DOG OWNERS VETERINARY GUIDE
AP-927

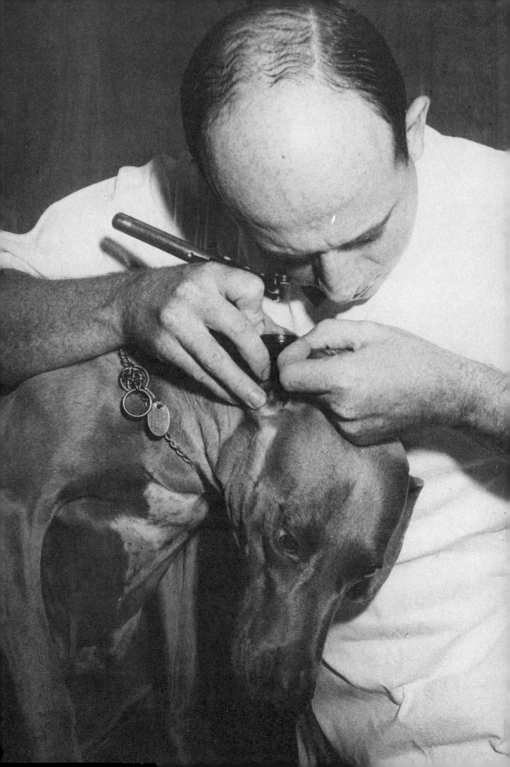

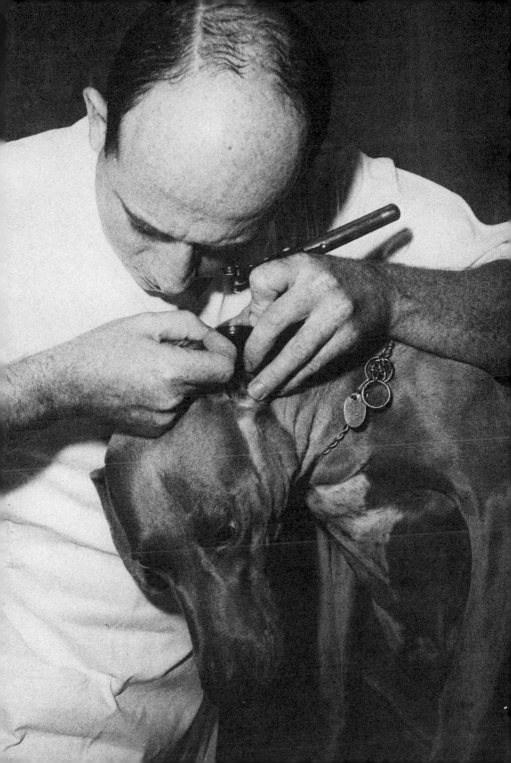

Accurate — Practical — Up-to-Date

The facts in this book are based on the most recent information set forth by America's foremost veterinarians. The book was edited by one of the nation's leading editors of veterinary literature, Dallas S. Burch, former official of the Bureau of Animal Industry, United States Department of Agriculture.

Illustration of the text by Eugene de L'horbe, unless otherwise indicated.

Dog Owner's
VETERINARY
GUIDE

By G. W. STAMM

Author of Veterinary Guide for
Farmers. Founder of Science Digest
and for ten years editor of that
magazine

Distributed in the U.S. by T.F.H. Publications, Inc., 211 West
Sylvania Avenue, PO Box 427, Neptune, NJ 07753; in England by
T.F.H. (Gt. Britain) Ltd., 13 Nutley Lane, Reigate, Surrey; in Canada
to the book store and library trade by Beaverbooks Ltd., 150 Lesmill
Road, Don Mills, Ontario M38 2T5, Canada; in Canada to the pet
trade by Rolf C. Hagen Ltd., 3225 Sartelon Street, Montreal 382,
Quebec; in Southeast Asia by Y.W. Ong, 9 Lorong 36 Geylang,
Singapore 14; in Australia and the South Pacific by Pet Imports Pty.
Ltd., P.O. Box 149, Brookvale 2100, N.S.W. Australia; in South Africa
by Valid Agencies, P.O. Box 51901, Randburg 2125 South Africa.
Published by T.F.H. Publications, Inc., Ltd, the British Crown Col-
ony of Hong Kong.

TABLE OF CONTENTS

Dog Owner's
VETERINARY
GUIDE

Can You Be Your Own Veterinarian?

YOU, AS A DOG OWNER, may be a successful surgeon or you may have no medical knowledge whatsoever. Dogs are owned by people in all walks of life.

But regardless of your background, there are many things concerned with your dog's health that you can learn to do. For example, you can learn to treat minor wounds, give medicines, provide proper food; you can rid your dog of fleas, mange and most kinds of worms. Other tasks, such as ear-cropping and tail-docking, require a little more skill. Still others can be performed only by someone with broad veterinary or medical knowledge.

Experience Is Important

Physicians and those in professions akin to the practice of medicine are of course familiar with the basic principles of veterinary medicine. Individuals such as laboratory workers, former sergeants in the Army Medical Corps and trained nurses have an advantage in experience and training over most people.

It boils down to this: Whether or not you can give your dog proper medical attention depends upon your knowledge, your experience and your native ability. Some people with little book knowledge have a natural "know-how" in matters of this kind.

Be Sure Before You Go Ahead

Those who are not familiar with the elements of diagnosis and treatment, are urged to proceed with care. Some of the chapters in the back of the book are designed primarily to interest those who already have some knowledge of veterinary or medical practice, for example, the chapters on how to give an anesthetic and how to set a broken bone.

No normal adult will unnecessarily injure or cause pain to a dumb animal. Certainly no one wants to take the chance of killing a pet. Always see your veterinarian when you have doubts as to whether you can successfully treat your sick or injured dog.

Finding Out What's Wrong

IT'S USUALLY easy to tell when your dog is sick. But sometimes it's not so easy to tell what's wrong with him.

People often say it's hard to diagnose the ailment of a dog because he can't tell you which part of his body hurts. Such people should remember that although a dog can't tell you about his symptoms, neither does he give you a lot of false information about them. He's not like a small boy who plays sick to keep from going to school or like some old gal who enlarges upon her ailments to get sympathy or attention.

The difficulties of diagnosis lie in the fact that many diseases have some symptoms in common and that some diseases do not always have the same symptoms. Fever, loss of appetite and lack of energy, for example, occur with many maladies, and distemper has varying symptoms depending upon which parts of the body are affected.

Dogs Have Their Off Days

Dogs, like people, have their off days. At times, for no apparent reason, they don't feel quite so well as usual. So, if some day your dog just likes to lie around, wait a while before you decide that he has something the matter with him.

Another thing: dogs that have the run of the neighborhood often have minor stomach ailments. They may vomit even though otherwise in the best of health. No doubt people would also have more stomach trouble if they went around gnawing old bones or eating scraps of rotten meat that have been lying in the dirt. So don't take your dog's disordered stomach too seriously unless, of course, it persists.

The Different Kinds of Symptoms

From a practical standpoint, there are three kinds of symptoms: those that can be readily observed; those that can be determined by use of simple methods, such as taking the temperature or the pulse; and those that can be found only by use of laboratory methods — microscopic examinations, chemical tests, and so on.

The Nature of Fever

Fever is one of the earliest signs of an acute disease caused by microbes. The principal other causes of fever are severe injuries and tumors.

The normal rectum temperature of a dog ranges between 101 and 102 degrees Fahrenheit, but since dogs cannot lose heat through perspiration as do many other animals, their temperature rises rapidly with exercise.

A Greyhound after a race has been known to have a temperature of 105 degrees. Similarly when the temperature of the surrounding air reaches 80 degrees or more, the temperature of a dog tends to rise.

The digestion of food causes a slight rise in temperature. A bitch has a higher temperature than normal towards the end of pregnancy. Such increases in temperature are natural but must be taken into consideration when determining whether fever is present.

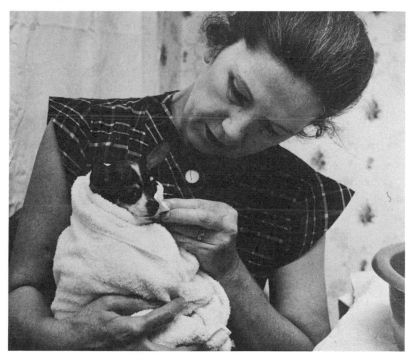

It's usually easy to tell when a dog is sick. But it's not so easy to tell what's wrong with him. Accurate diagnosis depends upon careful study of symptoms.

The symptoms of fever are an abnormal rise in temperature, loss of appetite, hot dry skin, increased thirst, digestive disturbances, more rapid heart beat and faster breathing. Chills often occur with the onset of fever when microbes or their toxins (poisons) are in the blood stream. Chills are commonly accompanied with a rise in hair coat and coolness of the skin.

A rapid rise in temperature of five or six degrees that soon returns to normal is less dangerous than a slow rise of three degrees that does not subside. One temperature reading is usually not enough for diagnostic purposes. Generally, readings should be taken twice a day and in acute cases four times a day.

How to Take the Temperature

To take the temperature of a dog, first make sure that the mercury in the thermometer has been shaken down into the bulb. Then grease the bulb end of the thermometer with vaseline or some other harmless lubricant. Push the thermometer, bulb end first, gently into the dog's rectum. Leave it there for at least three minutes before taking it out and reading the temperature.

The Pulse and What It Tells

The pulse tells how fast the heart is beating. It also reports the rhythm and strength of the beat. In this way it gives clues to the physical condition of an animal.

The pulse rate increases with fever, inflammation, hem-

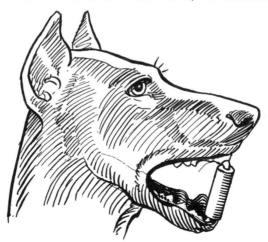

To keep a dog's mouth open for examination, drill a hole in each end of a piece of broomstick and insert it between the jaws.

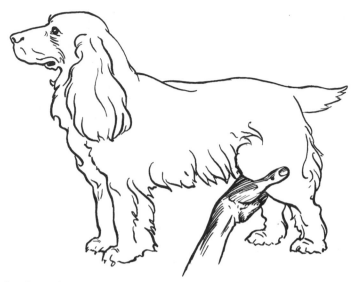

To take the pulse, rest a finger on the femoral artery which runs down the inner surface of a dog's hind leg.

orrhage, paralysis and diseases of the valves of the heart. The rate also increases with exercise, excitement, fear, hot weather, severe pain, and the digestion of food, but in such cases it rapidly returns to normal when these influences are no longer present.

In anemia and leukemia the pulse is usually weak. During collapse the pulse can hardly be felt. In meningitis and peritonitis the pulse is usually hard, that is, the artery feels hard or incompressible.

The normal pulse of dogs varies between 70 and 120 beats per minute, depending upon age and breed. In old animals and in large breeds, the pulse is generally slower than in young or small ones. Thus, the normal pulse of a healthy adult Great Dane might be 60 to 70, while that of an adult Pekingese might be as fast as 120. In both large and small dogs, the pulse becomes sluggish in old age.

A pulse of 120 in a large dog or 180 in a small one indicates that the animal is seriously ill.

How to Take the Pulse

The arteries — the blood vessels that lead away from the heart — all have a pulse and lend themselves to counting the heart beat. The artery most commonly used in taking the pulse

7

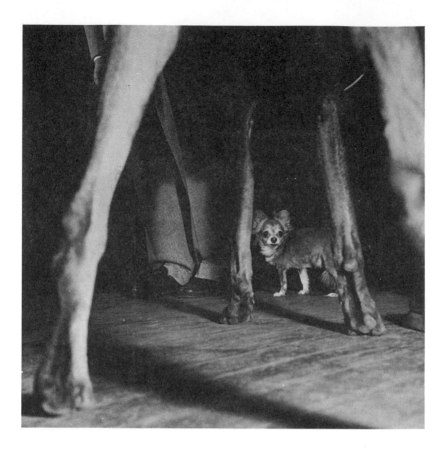

These dogs have the same normal body temperature but the normal pulse rate of the Chihuahua may be twice that of the Great Dane. In general, the smaller the animal, the faster the pulse.

of a dog is the femoral artery because it is comparatively large and easy to find. It runs down the inner surface of the hind leg and the best place for taking the pulse is where the artery comes out of the groin.

To take the pulse, roll the artery gently under a finger until you have found a good spot. Before you start to count, make sure that you can feel all beats plainly. Don't use your thumb for taking the pulse because it has a pulse of its own which you might mistake for that of the dog. It isn't necessary to count a full minute. Count for 30 seconds and multiply by two, or 15 seconds and multiply by four, if you prefer.

Diagnosis Is Often Difficult

Symptoms are, of course, not in themselves diseases. They merely indicate that disease is present. Diagnosis — the art of identifying a disease by its symptoms — is perhaps the most difficult subject in the practice of veterinary medicine. In most cases, treatment is comparatively simple, once the nature of the malady is definitely known.

Only through study and practice can a person become a good diagnostician. However, the following list of symptoms, together with the names of the diseases with which they are associated, will enable you to identify the more common ailments of dogs. It will also give you clues to which of the less common diseases might be present.

Some of the maladies listed are not dwelt upon elsewhere in this book because they are too rare or unimportant to warrant discussion in a volume of this size.

Common Symptoms and What They Indicate

Abdomen, Enlargement of — Abdominal dropsy (ascites.) Excessive fat. Hernia. Pregnancy. Distended bladder. Bloat. Enlargement of the spleen or liver. Tumor. Parasites in young puppies. Weakness of abdominal muscles in old dogs.

Abdomen, Tender — Acute dyspepsia. Acute gastritis. Foreign body perforating bowel. Poisoning. Tumors. Peritonitis.

Appetite, Abnormally large — Diabetes. Pregnancy. Beginning of heat period. Nursing (of bitches). (Ravenous appetite of growing puppies and of half-starved dogs is, of course, natural.)

Appetite, Depraved (Eating dirt, etc.)—Teething. Pregnancy. Lack of certain vitamins. Worms. Not enough salt in food.

Appetite, Lack of — Fever. Painful condition of teeth, mouth or throat. Overeating. Lack of certain minerals or vitamins. Parasites. Change in kind of food.

Breath, Foul — Tartar. Pyorrhea. Decayed or loose teeth. Ulcers along inside of cheeks. Constipation. Old age. Kidney disease. Cancer. Nose infections. Inflamed, spongy gums.

Breathing, Difficult (especially following exercise)—Pleurisy. Pneumonia. Heart trouble. Anemia. Heartworms.

9

Coughing — Bronchitis. Laryngitis. Pharyngitis. Pneumonia. Pleurisy. Asthma. Heart disease. Tracheitis. (Any or all of these ailments may occur during or following distemper). Worms. Hard pad disease.

Diarrhea — Improper diet. Worms. Coccidiosis. Nervousness. Poisoning. Rickets. Colitis. Extreme old age.

Gagging — Worms. Obstruction in throat. Tonsillitis. Hard pad disease.

Gums, Pale (anemia) — Hemorrhage (external or internal). Faulty diet. Starvation. Parasites. Piroplasmosis. Poisoning. Lack of sunlight. Stomach and intestinal disorders. Tumors. Wasting and malignant disease.

Hoarseness — Laryngitis. Pharyngitis. Tonsilitis. Obstruction in throat. Throat infections. Asthma.

Jaundice — Poisoning. Liver ailments. Leptospirosis. Piroplasmosis.

Muscular Spasms (convulsions) — Poisoning. Worms. Eclampsia. Diabetes. Encephalitis.

Nose, Running — Head cold. Distemper. Worms in nose. Salmon poisoning. Pneumonia.

Paralysis — Injured spine. Rabies. Distemper. Stroke.

Skin Disturbances — Mange, Eczema, Fleas, Acne. Alopecia.

Slobbering — Injuries to tongue, lips or mouth. Poison. Encephalitis. Insect bites. Splinters or other foreign bodies in mouth.

Swellings — Abscesses. Tumors. Dropsy. Heart trouble. Kidney disease. Goiter. Hernia. Leukemia. Bites of insects or snakes.

Thirst, Abnormal — Fever. Hemorrhage. Diarrhea. Kidney disease. Diabetes. Dropsy.

Tongue, Coated — Dyspepsia, Gastric catarrh. Distemper. Biliousness. Kidney diseases.

Trembling — Cold. Poison. Eclampsia.

Vomiting — Eating grass. Car sickness. Worms. Poisons. Strangulated hernia. Brain tumor. Kidney ailments. Peritonitis.

Weight, Loss of — Not enough food. Long illness. Diarrhea. Heart disease. Tuberculosis. Kidney ailment. Liver ailment. Arsenic poisoning. Diabetes. Tumors. Parasites.

The Truth About Distemper

DISTEMPER OF DOGS is a disease that appears suddenly and affects principally dogs between two months and one year old. While dogs of any breed may come down with distemper, those that are highly bred are more likely to get it than mongrels. Distemper is considered the worst of all dog ailments with the exception of rabies.

The disease is caused by a virus. It is highly contagious for dogs but other house pets and people are immune to it.

Dogs get the disease principally by way of the mouth, nose and ears. The virus may be spread by insects and worms may carry it in their bodies. Even before symptoms appear, the breath of a dog coming down with distemper may infect healthy animals.

Distemper can occur at any time of the year. The interval from the time of infection until symptoms appear is usually five days but may be anywhere from four days to 10 days. A dog that recovers from distemper is unlikely ever to have it again.

Symptoms

Distemper causes inflammation of the lining of the body, such as the inside of the mouth and nose and the lining of the intestines. It also sometimes causes pustules—pimples filled with pus—to appear on the skin.

Early symptoms are usually mild. There is a watery discharge from the nose and eyes, appetite falls off and the animal seems all tired out. The victim may vomit. It will shun the light as though light hurts its eyes. In some cases, dogs with distemper are giddy and have running fits during the first few days, but such symptoms soon disappear.

In about a week, a thick discharge comes from the nose and eyes. A dry hacking cough appears, nostrils become dry and the dog shivers. Thirst increases and temperature usually rises to between 103 and 105 degrees. Later the brain and spinal cord may be affected. This brings about nervous twitchings, convulsions and even paralysis.

Diarrhea usually occurs throughout the course of the disease. The stool is dark-colored and has a foul-smelling odor.

Distemper acts like the "flu." Many symptoms are similar. As in influenza, the disease breaks down the body resistance. Thus it paves the way for so-called secondary infections such as pneumonia, inflammation of the intestines (enteritis) or inflammation of the brain (encephalitis).

It is now known that the virus of distemper disappears from the blood a few days after symptoms are first noticeable. The disease is then prolonged principally by the secondary infections. Though the virus no longer appears in the blood, it still is present in other parts of the body. Later on in the course of the disease it often does a lot of damage to the internal organs.

Estimates vary as to the percentage of deaths among distemper patients. This is probably because the disease apparently differs in its seriousness from year to year. One authority says that much depends upon the breed. Among Bull Terriers 90 percent will recover while among other breeds such as Bloodhounds and Great Danes, only 10 percent will recover.

Animals that do not die from the disease may be left wholly or partially disabled. Some are deaf, blind or left with little or no sense of smell. Others have nervous muscle twitchings known as chorea or St. Vitus dance. Some undergo a complete change of personality though they seem all right physically. A few go insane.

The course of the disease is usually about a month but it may be as long as several months, depending upon the complications.

Distemper is often difficult to diagnose because symptoms vary in accordance with which organs are most affected, whether throat, lungs, digestive organs, nervous system or skin. Where it is known that there is distemper in the neighborhood or that a puppy has been exposed to the disease, it is likely that your dog has distemper if it shivers, sneezes, has diarrhea, partial loss of appetite and slight eye and nasal discharges.

Treatment

There is no cure for distemper. Once the symtoms have appeared, the disease will run its course regardless of medi-

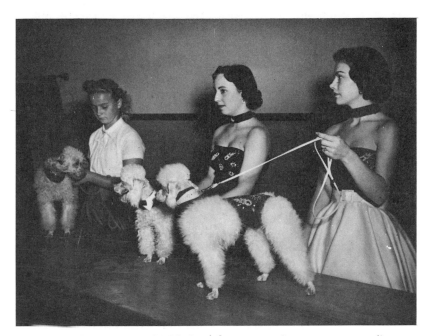

For some unknown reason highly bred dogs are much more apt to get distemper than are mongrels.

cines. Veterinarians sometimes inject immune serum to combat the disease but results are not uniform.

Dogs with distemper should be kept in clean, dry, well-ventilated quarters. They should be given small quantities of nourishing foods that are easily digested such as milk, eggs, raw beef and beef broth.

The discharge should be removed from the eyes often, otherwise the lids will become gummed together. Eyes may be bathed in a weak boric acid solution. Yellow oxide of mercury ointment, for sale at drug stores, may be applied to prevent sticking of eyelids. The discharge from the nose should also be removed. Vaseline or mentholatum may be applied to nostrils to keep them from cracking.

No way has been found to relieve the nervous derangements that often occur during and following distemper. The persistent twitching of the muscles frequently gets worse and worse until the muscles involved are paralyzed. There has, of course, been some success in treating the secondary diseases of distemper where these are recognized—pneumonia, for example.

Except in cold weather, the distemper virus lives only a short time outside the body of an animal. When premises are warm and dry, the virus is probably dead within a week after a victim of the disease has been removed. However it is best to wait at least three weeks before permitting an unvaccinated dog to occupy the premises. If it is necessary to use the premises sooner, a good safeguard consists in disinfecting them with a solution of lye, or cresol, or formaldehyde. Bedding and litter that might have become contaminated should be burned.

Prevention

Positive protection against distemper can be obtained through vaccination. There are a number of good ways to vaccinate. In one method a dose of vaccine is injected, followed in a week by a dose of living virus. Another method consists in injecting anti-canine-distemper serum and virus at the same time. A third method involves the use of a special virus that has been weakened by passing it through the bodies of a number of ferrets. When this so-called attenuated virus is injected into a dog, it causes a mild form of the disease which is followed by immunity. This is like vaccination against smallpox in human beings.

The necessary biologicals cannot be used safely and with proper skill by the general public. Nearly every veterinarian, however, can immunize your puppy by a number of methods and you will then have almost complete assurance that your dog will be safe from the dreaded distemper.

It is generally believed that puppies should not be immunized against distemper until they are at least three months old, otherwise the immunity may not last. To play safe, of course puppies can be vaccinated when very young and again later. Dogs to be vaccinated should be free from parasites and should otherwise be in good health.

Look Out for Infectious Hepatitis

INFECTIOUS HEPATITIS is a disease of dogs caused by a virus. It occurs in dogs of all ages but most often among young dogs. Puppies are the most apt to die from the disease.

The malady is believed to be spread principally by mouth since the virus is found in the saliva of infected animals. However the virus has also been found in the urine of dogs that have recovered from the disease, even six months after all other symptoms of the malady have disappeared.

It has been estimated that at least 75 percent of the older dogs are immune to hepatitis whereas nearly all puppies are susceptible. From this, authorities conclude that older dogs that are immune had a mild attack of the disease while still puppies—perhaps unnoticed at the time.

Until a few years ago, infectious hepatitis was not recognized as a separate ailment but was thought to be a form of distemper. Research at Cornell University, completed in 1951, showed that dogs can have distemper followed by infectious hepatitis or hepatitis followed by distemper, or they can have both diseases at the same time.

In other words there is no interference between the two ailments. In the past when an animal had two diseases at once, the malady was probably diagnosed as a severe form of distemper.

Symptoms

The word hepatitis means inflammation of the liver. First noticeable symptom of the disease is usually loss of interest in things. A dog, otherwise alert, withdraws from people and may hide in a dark corner. Appetite disappears and occasionally there is intense thirst. The head and neck may become swollen. Tonsils become enlarged.

Usually there is a watery discharge from the eyes that later becomes pus-like. The heart beats faster and the dog breathes rapidly. Vomiting and diarrhea may occur.

Temperature goes as high as 105° F. but subsides to normal, or below, before death. The disease reaches its height

15

in two to four days. There are no nervous symptoms as is the case with distemper. About ten percent of the infected animals die.

Of the dogs that recover, about one-third get a white film over one or both eyes, which may last from a few days to several weeks and then disappear.

Puppies with infectious hepatitis sometimes appear perfectly normal even though they have a high fever. They may run and play, yet the next morning be dead. Sometimes one or more puppies of a litter die while the others show no signs of the disease whatsoever.

Prevention

An antiserum is available which gives protection against the disease for about three weeks. This is often injected by veterinarians the day before dogs are taken on trips where they might become infected. A vaccine is also available which gives life-long protection against the malady. The vaccine is injected between the layers of the skin, a method known as intradermal injection.

Facts About "Hard Pad" Disease

HARD PAD disease was first recognized as a distinct malady in England in 1945 when supposedly reliable distemper vaccine failed to protect dogs against what appeared to be distemper. Since then hard pad disease has been identified in other countries, including hundreds of cases in the United States. It is caused by a virus.

The disease is said to be improperly named since the hard foot pads of affected dogs are only one of many symptoms. British veterinarians have called the malady demyelinating encephalitis and some Americans have called it paradistemper.

Symptoms

In the first stage of hard pad disease, the observable symptoms are almost identical with those of distemper. Like distemper, the disease runs its course despite medicinal treatment, and the death rate is high. It occurs more often in winter than in summer, while distemper shows no seasonal variation.

The disease can be distinguished from distemper in its sec-

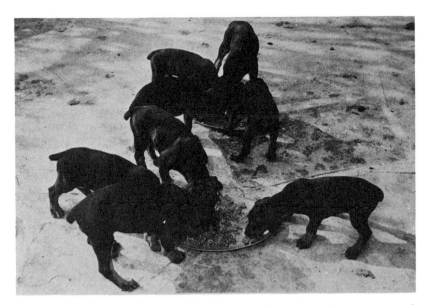

Distemper, infectious hepatitis and "hard pad" disease all strike puppies much more often than older dogs. The symptoms of the three diseases are similar.

ond stage. The foot pads become hard and enlarged as may the eyelids, tip of the nose, lips, hollow of the outer ears, the skin of the abdomen and the groin. Dark speckles appear on the abdomen and on the inner surface of the ears. Upon magnification, these pin-point areas show stubby enlargements of the hair roots.

In the third stage of the disease, the nervous system is affected. There are rapid involuntary biting movements together with a flow of frothy saliva. These so-called "champing fits" become more pronounced as the disease progresses. The peak of the malady is reached when affected dogs go into general convulsions. Animals reaching this stage usually die.

Treatment and Prevention

Treatment of sick dogs is the same as with distemper. A vaccine has been developed in England that gives protection against hard pad disease.

17

You Can Guard Against Rabies

RABIES, or hydrophobia, affects practically all warm-blooded animals, but it is principally a disease of dogs. It is caused by a virus and is spread through the saliva of an infected animal when it bites another. The virus attacks the nerves and gradually works its way to the brain.

Not every animal or person bitten by a rabid one will get the disease. Much depends upon whether the wound is deep or superficial and whether or not there is much bleeding. When there is a surface wound with a lot of bleeding, the virus is often washed away before it gets into the blood. Again it may get into the blood but may die before it becomes attached to a nerve.

Symptoms Slow to Appear

It takes from two weeks to as long as three months from the time an animal is bitten until symptoms appear. In dogs the first symptom of rabies may be a change in behavior. A dog becomes restless. Its disposition may change from friendly to snappy or the other way around.

Later, the animal may wander away for a few days. It may hide under a porch or in a dark corner. A change in the animal's voice may occur, a dismal bark and howl develop.

Symptoms vary somewhat in accordance with which parts of the nervous system and brain are attacked. Excitability, fits and various forms of paralysis may occur. Often the muscles become paralyzed and the animal is unable to drink.

Two Forms of the Disease

There are two distinct forms of the disease, depending upon which part of the nervous system is affected. In the dumb form, paralysis of the muscles is the most important symptom. The animal is not vicious. The muscles of its lower jaw are usually paralyzed and its mouth remains open. This symptom is sometimes mistaken for a bone in the throat and the dog owner often exposes himself to the disease by trying to remove the obstruction. It should be remembered that a

18

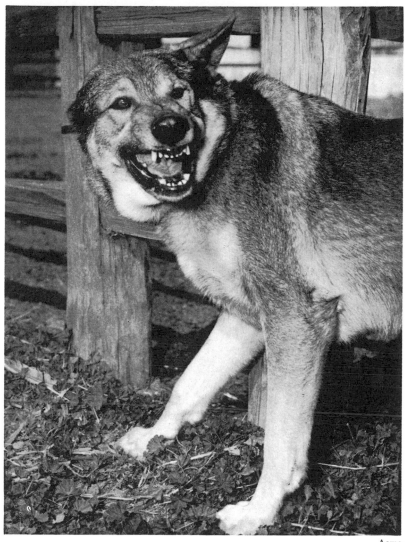

In the furious form of rabies, a dog is vicious and snaps at anything that gets in the way. Rabid dogs have been known to bite iron bars with such vigor that they broke their teeth.

dog with a bone in its throat will usually make efforts with its paws or otherwise to remove it, but a dog with rabies will not.

In the furious form of rabies, the dog roams for quite a

distance, is vicious and snaps at anything that gets in the way. If kept in a cage the dog may snap at the bars with such vigor that he breaks his teeth. No matter what form the disease takes, the victim dies within three to seven days after symptoms appear.

For an animal to infect another with rabies through a bite, it must of course itself be infected. But since the virus has been reported to be in a dog's saliva eight days before symptoms appear, a dog that bites should be confined for two weeks to make sure that it does not have rabies. Otherwise the public and other dogs may be exposed to the rabid dog's bite.

Prevention and Treatment

In England and a number of other countries, rabies has been completely wiped out. The same thing could be done here with proper control—by enforcing the laws covering stray dogs, and so on. Rabies can be prevented in dogs by means of vaccination, a job that is of course in the hands of veterinarians.

If you are bitten by a dog where there is the least suspicion of rabies, you should notify your doctor or the public health authorities at once. The Pasteur treatment started in time makes practically certain that the disease will not develop. The brains of dogs that presumably die of rabies are examined in public health laboratories to determine whether death was actually caused by the disease.

Feeding for Good Health

THOSE WHO are supposed to know, don't agree on what constitutes a balanced ration for dogs. Naturally the meat packers would like to have dogs eat mainly meat, and other food manufacturers highly recommend a ration made up largely from grains.

But how about the veterinarians and the kennel men? Why can't they agree, either among themselves or with each other?

One school of thought holds that a dog's teeth and digestive tract show that he is, and always has been, a meat eater. Another group says that dogs have depended upon people for so many centuries that their food habits have changed; their ration should consist principally of carbohydrates.

Both sides can produce evidence to prove their claims. Alaskan dogs thrive for long periods on meat and fat alone. On the other hand, research men have kept dogs in good health on diets containing no meat whatsoever.

To most dog owners, the matter of feeding is not merely a question of whether their dogs stay alive. They want their dogs to be good companions and they want the dogs to enjoy themselves. After all, why shouldn't a dog lead what politicians call "the more abundant life"?

The Necessary Foods

Physiologists agree that for vigorous health, dogs and other

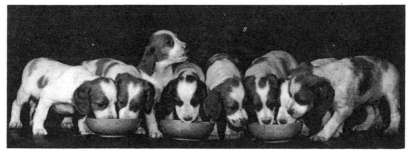

Jay Oppenhuisen

Puppies should be provided with individual dishes for food, otherwise the stronger ones get much more to eat than the others.

21

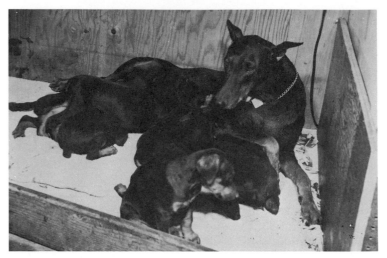

A nursing bitch may need twice as much food as ordinarily to make for the amount needed to produce milk.

animals must have proteins, carbohydrates and fats, minerals and certain vitamins. They also agree that dogs need some proteins of animal origin. The proteins in animal products are more complete in amino acids than those of vegetable origin. Amino acids are the building blocks of muscles and other tissues. The best food sources of them are first, milk and eggs, then liver and kidney, then muscle meat.

According to "Food and Life," a yearbook of the United States Department of Agriculture, the percentage of protein in a dog's diet may vary between wide limits. The most favorable proportion on an average for all dogs lies between 25 and 50 percent of the dry weight of the ration. Young dogs require considerably more per pound of weight than mature dogs. Pregnant and lactating bitches also require more.

Meats may be fed raw or cooked but not fried. Dogs usually don't like pork. There is danger in feeding them poultry because of the easily splintered bones. Canned fish and cooked fish with the bones removed are good protein feed. Puppies may start on a teaspoonful of ground or minced meat per day when about three weeks old. This may be increased to one or two tablespoonfuls at weaning time (six weeks) for medium-sized breeds.

The advantage of including carbohydrates in the diet is that they provide a cheap source of energy. Furthermore some carbohydrate is necessary for the utilization of fats. Boiled potatoes, boiled rice and other cereals are fed extensively to dogs. However, dogs cannot properly digest starchy foods unless they have been cooked.

Your Dog Needs a Lot of, Fat

For good health, dogs require much more fat than do human beings. Some authorities recommend a minimum of 15 percent fat in the diet. Forty percent can easily be tolerated. Sled dogs in the Far North eat as much as 70 percent.

Dogs like more salt in their food than do people. Some salt should be added to most feed. A dog should, of course, have all the clean water he wants.

Pregnant bitches should gradually be given more food as pregnancy advances and during this period the ration should consist of 65 to 75 percent animal products. During lactation, a bitch should have enough additional food to make up for that needed in producing milk. A pregnant or lactating bitch may need twice as much feed as one without these drains on her body resources.

Preparatory to weaning, the best food for puppies is cow's

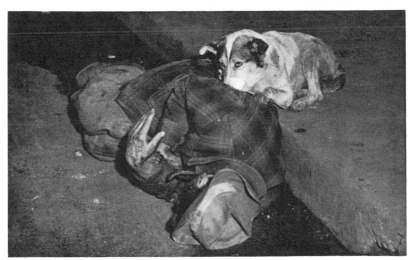

Men such as this one asleep in the gutter are generally not good providers for their dogs. Strangely, neither are some of the very rich; they pamper their pets with improper food.

Two Methods for Weighing a Dog

Make a loop of tape or rope and put it around the dog's neck. Then suspend the dog on the scale as shown below.

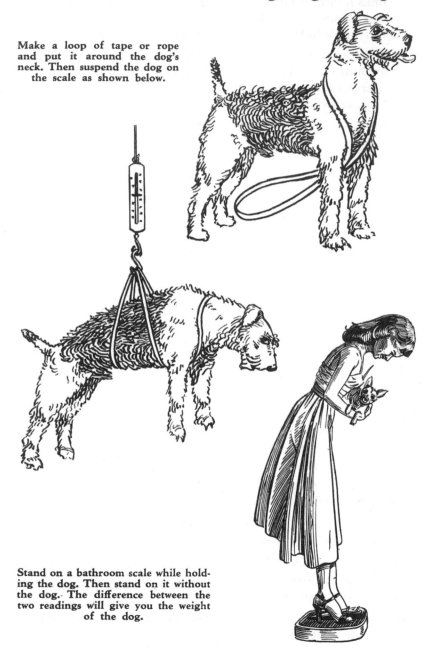

Stand on a bathroom scale while holding the dog. Then stand on it without the dog. The difference between the two readings will give you the weight of the dog.

milk. Immediately after weaning, puppies should be fed five or six times a day, gradually tapering off to two meals a day at one year of age. It may be advisable to include a small amount of cod-liver oil in the ration, particularly during the winter.

The amount of food needed by a dog depends upon age, size, and amount of exercise. For dogs getting moderate exercise, the approximate weight per day of feed required, including moisture, is as follows:

Weight in Pounds	Daily feed, Pounds	Weight in Pounds	Daily feed, Pounds
1	$\frac{1}{8}$	75	$3\frac{1}{4}$
10	$\frac{3}{4}$	100	4
25	$1\frac{1}{2}$	150	$5\frac{1}{4}$
50	$2\frac{1}{2}$	225	7

Rules of Feeding in Brief

Don't overfeed or underfeed your dog. Overfeeding makes dogs lazy and may induce sickness and impotency. Underfeeding makes dogs listless and may also induce sickness. Overfeeding is worse than underfeeding.

Keep a puppy growing steadily and uniformly but not too fast. To do this, keep him a trifle hungry. Feed him often but a little at a time.

Avoid giving your dog food that is too hot, too cold, highly seasoned or fried. Avoid sweet foods.

Don't take your dog's appetite as a guide to his feed requirements. Many dogs overeat when they have a chance. Through force of habit, they often shun foods that are good for them. If your dog is obstinate about eating some important food, let him starve for a day or so. He'll come around, all right.

Keep feeding and drinking utensils scrupulously clean.

Watch out for food allergies. Feed that is tolerated by one dog may cause digestive and other disturbances in another.

Exercise your dog at least once a day.

Feed at regular intervals.

Don't feed a ration containing a large amount of sloppy feeds. Avoid excessively bulky foods. particularly for puppies, hard-working dogs, and pregnant and lactating bitches.

Suspect internal parasites if your dog loses weight despite an adequate ration.

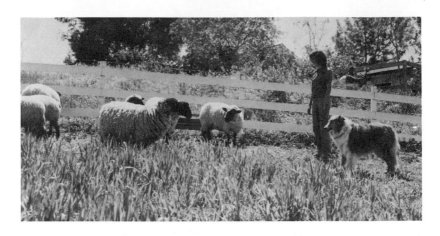

Dogs at work naturally require more food than others. But a dog's appetite should not be taken as a guide to his food requirements. If given a chance, a great many dogs will overeat.

Don't feed a dog immediately before or after he is exercised. A rest period for at least half an hour before and after eating aids digestion.

Don't force your dog to eat if he happens to go "off feed" for a day. This sometimes happens to animals in the best of health.

Feed and exercise your dog in such a way that he has bright clear eyes, a good coat and an abundance of energy. These are the sure signs of health.

Feed a mature dog a light meal in the morning and a heavier one in the afternoon or evening. A night watch dog, however, should have his heavier meal in the morning.

Dogs Need Minerals and Vitamins

THE ANCESTORS OF THE DOG got their food almost entirely by killing and eating other animals. They ate not only the flesh but also the livers and intestines of their prey, including the contents of these organs. They gnawed the bones and ate the marrow.

Thus the diet of those early animals consisted mostly of meat but was rich in vitamins, minerals and fat.

Today the dog eats what his master gives him. Usually this is good but sometimes it isn't.

Vitamin D and Rickets

Rickets is a disease generally of puppies or young dogs caused by lack of calcium or phosphorus or by failure of the body to absorb these elements properly. When they are in the diet but not absorbed, the cause is usually lack of vitamin D, which appears to regulate the absorption of the minerals.

Signs of rickets are lack of energy, arched back, crouched stance, knobby bone joints, bowed legs and flabby muscles. In more severe cases, the long bones of the legs fail to grow, become soft and are easily broken. Development of teeth is also retarded.

In dogs, it has been shown that rickets is usually of the low-phosphorus kind. The phosphorus in the food is not taken up by the body because the animal is not getting enough vitamin D.

Bonemeal amounting to one or two percent of the ration will provide enough calcium and phosphorus for puppies of small breeds. This should be fed to them if the rest of the diet is lacking in these elements. Puppies of larger breeds should have bones and milk in addition to the bonemeal.

The ultraviolet rays of the sun—greater in the summer—cause vitamin D to form in the bodies of animals. A so-called sun-lamp will do the same thing.

Where dogs, particularly puppies, are not exposed to ultraviolet light, whether in sunlight or otherwise, they should be

27

provided with vitamin D in their food. Good sources of this vitamin are fish-liver oils, eggs, salmon, sardines and butter. Fair sources are liver, cream and whole milk.

Anemia from Improper Diet

Anemia occurs when the blood does not contain enough hemoglobin, the red part that carries the oxygen to the tissues and carries away the carbon dioxide. The lack of hemoglobin may be because each red cell does not contain enough of it, because there are not enough red cells, or because there is lack of blood as in the case of a hemorrhage.

The ailment may be brought on by infectious diseases, hemorrhage, internal parasites, poisoning or improper diet. Nutritional anemias occur when the diet does not contain enough of the elements necessary to build hemoglobin properly. Nutritional anemia is commonly caused by insufficient iron, copper, B vitamins or underfeeding of proteins of animal origin.

Even a mild case of anemia is easy to recognize. The inside

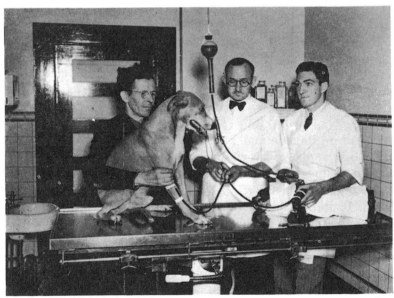

Acme

Veterinarians sometimes give an anemic dog a blood transfusion. Canine blood is typed, but unlike human beings, dogs apparently do not suffer any ill effects if given blood that differs from their own.

surface of the eyelids, the gums, and other mucous membranes are pale. In more severe cases, the pulse rate increases, breathing becomes faster and the animal tires easily.

Iron and copper are needed to form hemoglobin. Iron becomes part of this substance. Copper is needed only in very tiny amounts. It doesn't form part of the hemoglobin but its presence is necessary for the absorption of iron.

The iron requirements of a normal dog are met in a ration containing as little as ten percent of meat scraps. Excellent sources of iron are liver, kidney, red meat and egg yolk. Food that contains enough iron also contains enough copper to maintain health.

A bitch needs more iron during pregnancy so should be allowed a more liberal allowance of foods that are rich in iron. A normal puppy is born with a reserve store of iron. This is largely used up during the suckling period when the principal food is milk. The loss of iron is made up later when iron-rich foods are added to the milk diet.

Anemia is also brought on by deficiency of vitamin B_6. This is relieved by feeding fresh liver, liver concentrates or liver extracts.

Eclampsia, a Disease of Nursing Bitches

Eclampsia is a disease that affects nursing bitches, especially those with large litters. It occurs most often between a few days and several weeks after whelping, but may occur shortly before or during that time.

The malady appears suddenly. Symptoms are panting, excitement, shivering, and the appearance of a fit. The animal may fall on its side and kick violently, muscles become tense, breathing rapid, pulse rate is increased. The animal remains conscious during an attack. If not attended to, she may die.

Eclampsia is brought on by lack of enough calcium in the blood. It occurs mainly during the nursing period because of the large amount of calcium needed for the milk of the bitch.

Treatment consists in injecting calcium gluconate into a vein. The dose is one cubic centimeter of a 20 percent solution for each two pounds of weight. This usually brings recovery within 15 minutes. The bitch should be placed in warm quarters and not allowed to nurse her puppies for some time after recovery.

Lack of Vitamin A

Often a diet supplies nearly all but not quite enough vitamin A for the needs of the body. In such cases symptoms of a deficiency are very difficult to detect.

Perhaps the most easily recognized symptom of severe lack of vitamin A is an eye disease called xerophthalmia in which the eyeball becomes first watery, then dry and then lusterless and the eyelids become inflamed. Other symptoms are night blindness, loss of weight, rough coat, scaly skin, and stunted growth among puppies. If the disease is allowed to progress, permanent blindness may result.

The ailment is easily cured by addition of fish-liver oil or liver to the diet.

Vitamin B_1 and B_2 Deficiencies

Lack of vitamin B_1, also called thiamin, brings on a disease in dogs that resembles beriberi in humans. Symptoms are loss of appetite, vomiting, either diarrhea or constipation, swelling of the skin, muscular tenderness and inability to stand.

The malady is quickly cured by feeding an affected animal brewers yeast, meat, egg yolk, most fruits, or the outer portions of grains. Pork muscle contains about seven times as much thiamin as beef muscle. Since thiamin is easily destroyed by heat, about 80 percent of the vitamin may be lost during the canning of dog food.

Lack of vitamin B_2 has serious consequences but perhaps never occurs except when other vitamin B deficiencies are present also.

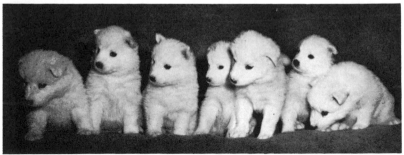

International

A normal puppy is born with a reserve store of iron. This is used up during the suckling period since milk does not contain enough to supply normal body requirements.

Blacktongue and Niacin

Blacktongue occurs principally in the southern states where the ration is similar to that which causes pellagra in people. This ration consists largely of corn meal, salt pork, cowpeas and sweet potatoes. Blacktongue is sometimes mistakenly called Stuttgart disease or canine typhus.

The disease is caused by lack of niacin which was formerly known as nicotinic acid.

Symptoms of blacktongue are lack of energy, loss of appetite and sometimes vomiting. The breath has a foul odor. The gums, the tongue and inside of the cheeks are reddened and have purplish-red areas. The inner surfaces of the cheeks and lips may be covered with ulcers and boils. Often there is constipation in the beginning, which is followed by diarrhea.

Death results if the disease is not relieved by feeding the affected animal niacin or liberal quantities of food containing the vitamin such as fresh liver, dried yeast, beef muscle, wheat germ, eggs, and milk.

Vitamin C

It is unnecessary to feed dogs fruit juice or green vegetables for them to have their supply of vitamin C. This vitamin is made in the dog's digestive tract from other foods.

Poisons and Their Antidotes

WHEN DOGS ARE POISONED it is nearly always by accident. They may eat garbage containing poisonous refuse, chew plants that have been sprayed or eat poisoned food intended for small animal pests, such as rats and moles.

Symptoms and First Aid

Symptoms of poisoning often resemble those of other diseases. They include trembling, abdominal pain, rapid shallow breathing, vomiting, convulsions, depression and coma. With some poisons, symptoms appear suddenly, with others the effect is cumulative—symptoms appear gradually as small quantities of the poison are eaten from day to day.

When poison is suspected, the animal should be given an emetic—something to make it vomit—immediately. A few minutes' delay may mean the difference between life and death of your pet.

Emetics

Emetics commonly given as antidotes for poison are the following:

Common Salt—Two teaspoonfuls in a cup of warm water.

Mustard—One tablespoonful in a cup of warm water.

Washing Soda—A piece the size of a hazelnut, pushed down the throat like a pill. Very large dogs require more.

Hydrogen Peroxide—This is perhaps the best emetic of all. Mix equal parts of hydrogen peroxide and water and force the animal to take one and one-half tablespoonfuls for each ten pounds of weight. Vomiting should occur in a few minutes.

After giving the emetic, call your veterinarian. If you know the source of the poison, you will find the antidote printed on the label. Otherwise your veterinarian will have to determine the kind of poison by the symptoms and employ the antidote for it. If you can't reach a veterinarian, you'll have to do the best you can to find out what kind of poison the dog has eaten. Below is a list of the more common poisons, together with symptoms they cause, and their antidotes.

The Common Poisons

ARSENIC—Occurs in rat and insect poison (Paris green). Symptoms are loss of appetite, intense thirst, signs of pain in abdomen, vomiting, bloody diarrhea, depression, rapid breathing and complete collapse.

One antidote is Epsom salts. This should be followed by limewater, whites of raw eggs, or milk with white of raw egg. The recognized antidote, however, is a solution prepared from iron sulfate and magnesium oxide. This solution is obtainable in drug stores.

PHOSPHORUS—Present in rat and insect poisons. Poisoning usually develops slowly, sometimes taking several days. Common symptoms are extreme restlessness, apparent pains in stomach, vomiting of material with greenish-brown color, swelling of tongue, jaundice and weakness. The vomit glows in the dark.

There are two standard antidotes: copper sulfate with one

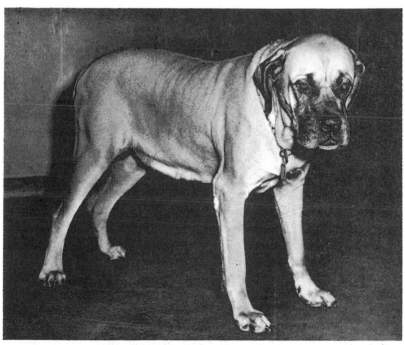

Acme

One sign of arsenic poisoning is intense mental degression. Other symptoms are loss of appetite, intense thirst and abdominal pains.

part to 50 parts of water, or one-tenth of one percent solution of potassium permanganate. First aid consists in giving equal parts of hydrogen peroxide and water as set forth above under emetics or three teaspoonfuls of milk of magnesia. Barley soup or oatmeal gruel may absorb some of the phosphorus. Never give castor oil or other laxative oils in this kind of poisoning.

LEAD POISONING—This usually comes from licking wet paint, or eating food or drinking water from old paint cans. It may also be eaten as lead arsenate used in sprays to kill insects.

Lead poisoning occurs in two forms. In the acute form the symptoms are trembling, labored breathing, colic, general weakness and coma. It results from consuming a large amount of a lead compound at one time. In the chronic form which occurs when small quantities of lead are taken over a long period, the principal symptom is bluish discoloration at the margin of the gums. Chronic lead poisoning is rare among dogs.

The antidote is Epsom Salts or Glauber salts, two teaspoonfuls to a glass of warm water. Raw white of egg and milk may also be given to relieve irritation of intestines.

STRYCHNINE—Dogs are much more sensitive to strychnine poisoning than people. The small amount contained in some cathartics, harmless to human beings, often severely poisons a dog. Strychnine is contained in some rodent poisons.

Symptoms are spasmodic twitching of the muscles, convulsions, and the inability of the animal to stand. The jaw becomes locked, eyes protrude, head and tail are drawn upward. Repeated convulsions are usually followed by death. Prompt treatment is important.

A powerful emetic should be given at once, such as a hypodermic injection of apomorphine. If this is not available, use emetics mentioned at beginning of this chapter. Spasms should be relieved with sedatives such as phenobarbital or Nembutal.

FOOD POISONING—Dogs that run loose and obtain part of their food from refuse and garbage cans may get food poisoning, although this rarely happens. Dogs are not nearly so sensitive to this form of poisoning as are human beings.

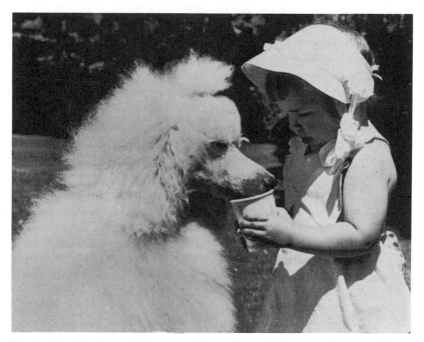

Nearly all poisonings of dogs occur by accident. Seldom are they traceable to revenge or other motives.

The poison is usually produced by bacteria acting on meat, either as scraps or complete carcasses. Symptoms include vomiting, bloody diarrhea, abdominal pains and general weakness.

Treatment consists in removing the poisonous material from the digestive tract as soon as possible. This can be done by means of emetics as described on page 32, or use of a stomach pump. After the stomach has been emptied, intestines should be cleared of the poison by means of a purgative or enema.

ACIDS—The symptoms of acid poisoning are similar to those of lead poisoning, often with excessive flow of saliva. Onset is rapid. The breath and vomit sometimes give a clue as to kind of acid present.

The antidotes for acids are sodium bicarbonate, chalk and water, or large doses of milk of magnesia. Crushed egg shell or plaster may also be given.

Hydrocyanic acid is about the only acid that occurs in nature in poisonous amounts. It is contained in wild choke-cherries, wild black cherries and in laurel leaves. Hydrocyanic acid is also known as prussic acid.

This poison acts so rapidly that when symptoms are noticed it is usually too late to do anything about it. When animal does not die, treatment consists of giving two tablespoonfuls of corn syrup.

ALKALIES—These occur in cleaning preparations such as sink cleaners. Antidote consists in giving an emetic as described on page 32, followed by several tablespoonfuls of vinegar or lemon juice.

DDT—This occurs in flea powders and bug poisons. In addition to general symptoms of poisoning, DDT causes muscular twitching.

To rid the system of the poison, an emetic should be followed by an enema. There is no known antidote for the drug.

Worms and How to Get Rid of Them

SEVERAL hundred different kinds of parasites attack dogs, most of them, however, doing little harm. Among the harmful internal parasites are the worms known by veterinarians as helminths.

Many of the helminths have complicated life histories. From eggs to adults they sometimes change their body forms several times and they may live parts of their lives inside the bodies of insects or other small animals.

It is practically impossible for a dog to lead a normal life without having some worms. But only when animals are heavily infested are the effects really serious. Puppies suffer the greatest damage from worms. In some strange way, older dogs become resistant to the effects of most kinds of worm parasites.

Nature has created a nice balance between parasites and their hosts. Nature says to the parasites. "Go ahead. Eat and drink your fill but not too much. If you do, you'll kill your host and then you'll die also."

Large Roundworms, or Ascarids

LARGE INTESTINAL roundworms, or ascarids, that infect dogs are five to eight inches long when full grown. Their eggs can be seen only with the aid of a microscope. Two kinds of roundworms commonly affect dogs and their life histories are nearly alike.

After being passed in the stools of dogs, the eggs generally become infective in two or three weeks. In the infective stage, each egg contains a tiny coiled worm known as an embryo. While in this stage, the embryo can live for years, waiting to be picked up by an animal.

A dog may pick up eggs on a piece of meat dragged in the dirt. A puppy may swallow eggs that were lodged on its mother's teats. When the eggs reach the intestines, the shells are digested and the embryos are released. An embryo released from its shell is called a larva.

The larvae of one kind of roundworm, *Toxascaris canis*, dig through the walls of the intestines, enter the blood stream, are carried to the liver and thence to the lungs. As they accumulate, they make the animal cough. In this way the larvae are swallowed and return to the intestines. Here they settle down and become full-grown in about two months. The sexes then mate and the females lay numerous eggs. This type of roundworm is particularly injurious to puppies.

Another kind of roundworm common among dogs is called *Toxascaris leonina*. Its larvae burrow deeply into the wall of the small intestines where they increase in size for about ten days. Then they emerge and remain in the hollow of the intestines until they die of old age or are killed by means of drugs.

Symptoms

While in the intestines, roundworms rob their hosts of nourishment. The most common symptoms of roundworm infection are unthriftiness, digestive disturbances and bloating. The hair coat is without luster and the breath may have a peculiar sweetish odor.

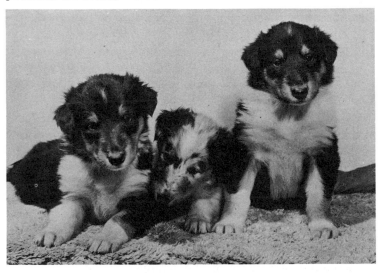

When one puppy of a litter is dewormed while another is not, the result is a marked difference in body growth.

Infested puppies may have potbellies, anemia, and temperatures below normal. Often there is diarrhea. Sometimes many worms form a mass of coils that obstruct the intestines so completely that the animal dies.

Perhaps the greatest damage done by roundworms is to lungs. The larvae puncture the tiny vessels in the lungs and weaken the tissues so that many animals get pneumonia.

Prevention

Use only clean containers for food and water. Bitches should be dewormed, where necessary, before breeding. So far as possible, puppies should be kept away from contaminated grounds. Teats of nursing bitches should be washed whenever they may have been exposed to worms.

No chemical treatment of premises will destroy the eggs of large roundworms, whipworms, lungworms or esophageal worms. Disinfectants will not penetrate the shells. Direct sunlight will kill eggs during the summer but the eggs survive a cold winter even when lying on top of the ground.

Treatment

The drug to use to get rid of roundworms depends upon the age of the dog. In young puppies, it is important that all worms be killed and removed from the digestive system. If the worms remain in the intestines and decay, they form poisons that may kill a puppy.

Living worms cannot be removed from the intestines through use of ordinary laxatives because the worms cling to the walls with great strength. Laxatives will, of course, remove dead worms.

With puppies, the stool should be examined to make sure that treatment is necessary. Even puppies three weeks old may have worms which they got before birth from the blood of the mother. Roundworms are whitish to yellowish and are pointed at both ends. They tend to curl up while alive but straighten out when dead. Ordinarily puppies should not be dewormed before they are weaned.

The best treatment for puppies is tetrachlorethylene (tetrachlor-ethyl-ene). It should be given in capsules, one-tenth cc to each pound of weight of the puppy.

It is extremely important that puppies be given nothing to

eat for 20 hours before treatment. The drug combines with any fat that may be in the food. When this happens, the drug is absorbed into the system with the fat. When the drug reaches the liver, the puppy often dies. Even a spoonful of milk in the stomach is dangerous.

The drug should be followed in an hour by a teaspoonful of milk of magnesia. Two hours after the puppy may be given food. Never use an oily laxative while tetrachlorethylene is in the digestive tract.

Tetrachlorethylene undergoes a change and may become poisonous unless it is kept in a cool dark place. In some animals it causes dizziness and unconciousness, but these effects are only temporary. The animal recovers of its own accord in a short time.

The drug can also be used in deworming adult dogs if the same precautions are taken. But a drug widely used and less dangerous is N butyl chloride. The dose is one cc for each ten pounds of weight. Its advantage over tetrachlorethylene is that it is safer. It doesn't have any bad reactions if given in proper doses and it does not combine with fat that may be present. The animal to be treated should be fasted and given a laxative just as when tetrachlorethylene is used. However, any good laxative may be used even though it contains fat.

Since these drugs do not reach the roundworms that may be in the blood or lungs, treatment should be repeated in two weeks. By that time such worms will have taken up residence in the intestines where they can be killed.

Esophageal Worms

ESOPHAGEAL worms of dogs are red and are usually coiled in a spiral. Females are about a half-inch to four inches long and males are about half that long. They occur commonly in dogs in the southern states.

Dogs become infected with the worms by swallowing dung beetles containing the infective larvae, or by eating small animals which in turn have eaten such dung beetles—rats, for example. The larvae are released in a dog's stomach and in a roundabout way some of them reach the dog's esophagus, the canal that extends from the throat to the stomach. They may

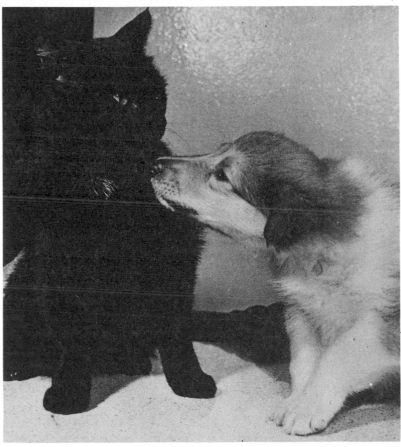

This fine fellow thinks he's pretty smart but he'd better watch out. Some of the worms and fleas that infest alley cats also relish dog meat.

also lodge in nearby parts. In their travels, the larvae damage blood vessels, particularly the aorta, the principal artery of the body.

Upon reaching the esophagus or nearby parts, the worms form tumors which may contain as many as 30 individuals. The tumors that open into the esophagus may exude a milky fluid that contains eggs and worms in various stages of development. The eggs pass out with the dog's stool. Later they are taken into the bodies of dung beetles.

Symptoms

Symptoms depend somewhat upon the location and size of the tumors. If they are in the esophagus, they cause difficult swallowing, vomiting and loss of weight. If the tumors press against the windpipe or lung, they may cause coughing, difficult breathing and suffocation. Sometimes they weaken the aorta so that it ruptures and the dog bleeds to death.

Treatment

Treatment consists in giving the affected dog hydrogen peroxide. This should be diluted to 1½ percent, just half the drug store strength. The peroxide should be poured into the dog's mouth so that it runs slowly down the throat. This will cause the dog to vomit. Thus the worms will be reached twice by drug—on the way down and on the way up. The peroxide should be given on an empty stomach, that is, three or four hours after the dog has eaten.

Whipworms

THE DOG WHIPWORM is shaped like a tiny whip. It is usually about two inches long—seldom longer than three inches. The body of the worm is no thicker than a heavy sewing thread. The front end is even more slender than the rest of the body and comprises about three-quarters of the length.

Whipworms live in the large intestines, and in the cecum.

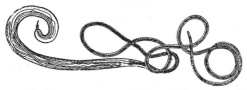

An adult whipworm is between two and three inches long. These worms are very common in dogs in the United States but usually do very little harm.

This is the portion of the intestines which corresponds to the appendix of humans, also known as the blind gut. The worms attach themselves within the cecum by sewing the slender ends of their bodies into the walls.

When infective eggs are swallowed by a dog, they hatch in the small intestines and then move on to the cecum and large intestines. They are found in the latter place only with heavy infestation and when the animal has not been given medicines to kill other worms.

The eggs of the whipworm pass out with the stool and become infective in from three weeks to several months. Dogs acquire the larvae by swallowing the eggs when the eggs are in the infective stage of development. It may take as long as three months from the time the eggs enter the intestines until the mature whipworms start to lay eggs.

Symptoms

In mild infestations, whipworms seem to do no particular harm. In more severe cases, symptoms include digestive disturbances, diarrhea, loss of weight, nervousness and fits.

Whipworms do not suck blood like hookworms, yet they sometimes cause anemia. Authorities believe that whipworms produce toxins, or poisons, which bring on anemia.

Prevention

Stools of infected animals should be removed promptly, and where practicable contaminated soil should be removed to a depth of several inches and replaced with clean sand.

Whipworms cannot be killed by ordinary disinfectants but direct sunlight will kill them during the summer. They cannot endure strong ultraviolet light.

Cellars and other damp places that have become contaminated may be disinfected by using a flame torch. An ordinary blow torch will also serve the purpose but of course takes longer than when a flame torch is used.

Treatment

Any drug that kills other worms will also kill the whipworm. The trouble is that whipworms lodge in the blind gut where you can't always kill them by ordinary deworming methods. Larger doses of drugs are usually necessary.

The drug generally used is N butyl chloride in doses three times as strong as recommended for other worms. (See page

40) this will generally remove most of the whipworms.

A dog should be given no food for 24 hours before treatment, otherwise the drug will be diluted and won't work as well. Before being dosed, the dog should be given something to keep him from vomiting. (See index for "Car Sickness").

Unless roundworms are also present it is not necessary to give a physic following treatment with N butyl chloride. Food may be given one hour after treatment. The treatment may be repeated after a week if the first one is unsatisfactory. N butyl chloride is contained in medicines sold by pet supply dealers.

Tapeworms

SEVERAL KINDS of tapeworms infect dogs. Some spend part of their life cycle in fleas and lice, others live part of the time in other mammals—in rabbits, for example. A few kinds of tapeworms require two hosts. They may live part of their lives in crayfish and another part in the bodies of fish before taking up their abode in dogs. Tapeworms may be anywhere from less than one-quarter inch to 16 feet long.

The tapeworm most common in dogs is called the *Dipylidium caninum.* It grows to be about a foot long. It spends part of its life in the body of a louse or flea. Dogs become infected when they swallow these vermin.

Symptoms

When only a few tapeworms are present, the animal suffers no apparent injury. In some cases, even dogs that are heavily infested are without observable symptoms. In other cases, however, animals have a tendency to vomit, they have digestive disturbances and are generally restless.

House pets with tapeworms are often a nuisance because the segments are frequently passed by the animals unintentially and soil housefurnishings. These segments are sometimes wrongly called pinworms. The passing of the segments sometimes irritates a dog's rectum in which case it will scratch itself by sitting down and dragging itself along by the forefeet. The presence of worm segments in a dog's stool naturally indicates that the dog has tapeworms. But the absence of segments does not necessarily mean that the dog is without them. Segments are not always passed in each stool.

Prevention and Treatment

There's no way to insure dogs against getting tapeworms but chances are less if dogs are kept from eating uncooked rabbit meat and fish, and are kept free of fleas and lice.

The most widely used drug for ridding dogs of tapeworms is arecoline hydrobromide, contained in patent medicine. The drug will completely remove the more common tapeworms within 45 minutes. The dog should be given no food for 15 to 18 hours before being dosed. Size of the dose is indicated on the label and should be strictly followed.

Hookworms

THREE KINDS of hookworms infect dogs. They all look alike except under the microscope and all have about the same life histories. None of them grow to be more than five-eighths of an inch long.

Females produce an enormous number of eggs, invisible to the naked eye. These pass out in the stool and generally hatch

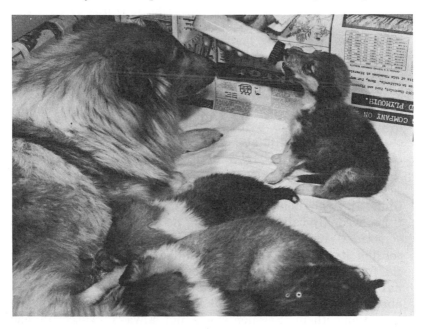

Puppies may get roundworms and hookworms before they are born. This is one of the reasons why pregnant bitches should always be dewormed.

45

in three to six days. Tiny young hookworms, or larvae, shed their skins several times over a period of about two weeks before reaching the infective stage.

Hookworms infect dogs, either through the mouth or through the skin. If they burrow through the skin into the blood stream, they soon reach the lungs. They are then coughed up, swallowed and thus reach the intestines. When hookworms are swallowed with contaminated food or water, they go directly to the intestines. Whichever way they get there, after reaching the intestines, the hookworms molt two more times and start to produce eggs in three to six weeks.

Hookworm eggs may appear in the stool of a puppy only 13 days old. This is because the puppy was infected before it was born.

The head end of a hookworm is curved upward. The mouth of the so-called common dog hookworm, *Ancylostoma caninum*, which is widely distributed, has three pairs of large curved teeth. Another, *Ancylostoma braziliense,* which occurs in warm climates, has one pair of large and one pair of small teeth. The third kind, *Uncinaria stenocephala,* which lives mostly in the north, has a cutting plate on each side of the mouth.

Hookworms are blood suckers. They attach themselves to the walls of the intestines when feeding. A single worm may puncture the intestines many times in the course of a day, sucking blood and letting it ooze out of the wound after each feeding.

Symptoms

The most damaging result of hookworms is anemia, caused by the loss of blood. A pale color of a dog's gums reveals this condition at once. Other symptoms of hookworms are diarrhea, stools that contain blood, loss of weight and sunken eyes. Sometimes legs swell and the dogs have fits. Anemia always causes lack of energy. The worms sometimes affect the lungs, as with roundworms, but symptoms are not nearly so severe. With heavy infestations, hookworms may cause death.

Puppies and young dogs are more susceptible to hookworm disease than older ones. The effects become less severe with repeated infestations. Well fed animals are not nearly so susceptible to hookworm disease as undernourished ones.

Prevention and Treatment

Preventive measures should be the same as those used with roundworm disease, set forth on page 39.

Soil contaminated with hookworm eggs and larvae can be sterilized with strong salt brine. Prepare the brine by adding 1½ pounds of salt to a gallon of boiling water. Sprinkle this over the soil so as to saturate it to a depth of ½ to 1½ inches. One pint of brine is enough for 1 square foot of surface. Treatment should be repeated when rain has washed the salt away.

Medicinal treatment for hookworms is the same as that prescribed for roundworms. (See page 39)

Heartworms

IT WAS FORMERLY believed that heartworms occur almost exclusively in warmer climates but now it is known that they may occur anywhere. They are becoming more and more common in areas where mosquitoes are present.

Female heartworms are ten to 14 inches long and less than one-sixteenth of an inch thick. Males are about half this size. Most of them live in the right side of the heart, in the part known as the ventricle which pumps blood to the lungs.

Unlike hookworms, roundworms and whipworms, heart-

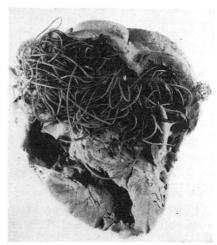

Heart of a dog, showing heavy infestation with heartworms. The disease is difficult to cure.

U.S.D.A.

worms do not develop from eggs. However the larvae will not grow into adult worms until they have passed through the bodies of insects, principally mosquitoes though sometimes fleas. The insects infect dogs by biting them.

The larvae are most abundant during the hours of darkness. If they are not sucked out by insects, they can live in the blood of a dog for several years. For this reason a dog that has apparently been cured of the disease may still be a source of infection if carrier insects are present.

It takes several months from the time an infected insect bites a dog until the worms appear in the heart. Little is known of the life of the larvae in the meantime.

The presence of heartworm disease varies with the age of the dog. The older the dog, the more he is apt to be infected. On the west coast of Florida, where the disease is common among dogs allowed to run at will, infections have been known to be as high as 37 percent of the animals between two and three years old and nearly 100 percent of those five years old and older.

Symptoms

Heartworms clog the heart so that the blood to the lungs does not flow freely. First symptoms usually appear after vigorous exercise. An infected animal tires easily, may gasp for breath and may even collapse. Coughing is common when the disease has been present a long time, the poor circulation may make the legs, abdomen and other parts of the body swell. Nervous symptoms, such as fear of lights, staring blankly at something, or convulsions, may develop.

Prevention and Treatment

Prevention consists in keeping animals from being bitten by mosquitoes and fleas. This of course is not easy. Animals kept in screened enclosures during the night, and at other times when mosquitoes are bad, are of course protected somewhat against the disease. Spraying dogs regularly with DDT is often practiced in areas where heartworm disease is common.

Treatment for heartworms is difficult and should be practiced only by a veterinarian or someone with similar technical skill. One drug used to treat the disease is Faudin, an anti-

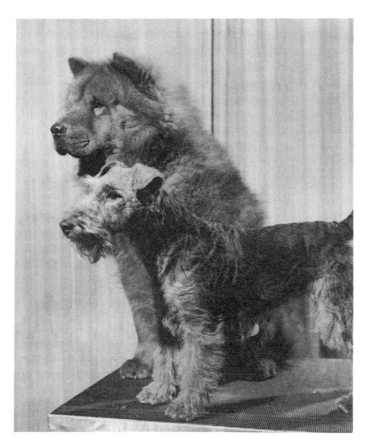

Unlike most internal parasites, heartworms do much more damage to older dogs than to young ones.

mony compound which is injected either into the veins or the muscles. A number of daily injections are made. Another drug used is called Caracide.

Even among veterinarians, the drugs in use against heartworms kill between five and ten percent of the dogs treated. Dangers in use of drugs lie in the fact that the dead heartworms clog the blood vessels that lead to the lungs and this sometimes completely cuts off circulation.

Latest Treatments for Mange

RED MANGE, also called demodectic mange, or follicular mange, is perhaps the most common skin disease of dogs. Until recent years it has also been the most difficult to cure.

It is caused by wormlike mites which live in the hair follicles and in some glands of the skin. The disease is most common among young animals, especially those with short hair.

The first symptom of red mange is the appearance of bald areas which are slightly reddened. The spots generally occur around the eyes, elbows, hocks and toes but may occur elsewhere. There is little or no itching at this time. Itching occurs later but is never so bad as in the case of sarcoptic mange.

After a while the hairless areas become larger until many of them merge. The skin becomes copper colored which accounts for the name "red" mange. In severe cases the skin may become gray or bluish. Inflammation sets in as a result of both the mites and the scratching. The skin becomes thick

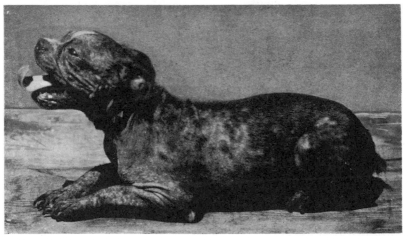

U.S.D.A.

A moderately severe case of red mange, also known as demodectic mange. This is the most common kind of mange and until recent years has been the most difficult to cure.

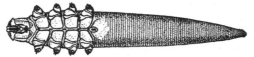

This is the mite that causes red mange. It is so small that it can be seen only under a microscope.

and raw. Germs usually infect the raw areas, form small pus pockets and give rise to unpleasant odors. The poisons produced by the microbes undermine the dog's health.

The disease runs a slow course, sometimes extending over a period of two years or more. Unless properly treated, a dog with red mange usually dies, although now and then a vigorous, well-fed animal recovers without medicinal treatment.

Red mange mites die in a few days if not on the body of a dog. For this reason premises do not remain contaminated for a long time after infected animals have been removed.

Diagnosis and Treatment

Red mange looks very much like some other skin diseases, including sarcoptic mange, fungus infections, acne and eczema. Positive diagnosis can be made only by examining skin scrapings or material from the pustules under the microscope. Even so, it sometimes takes several examinations to find the mites, particularly when the disease first starts.

Several good remedies are now available for treatment of red mange. Among them are rotenone, DDT, and benzine hexachloride. A refined form of benzine hexachloride, known as Lindane, is also widely used. Medicines for treatment of red mange are available at all pet-supply counters.

Sarcoptic Mange

THE MITES that cause sarcoptic mange are not much longer than one-hundredth of an inch. The adult females burrow into the upper layers of skin, where each lays 20 to 40 eggs. A male and female may have as many as 1,500,000 descendants in three months.

Sarcoptic mange affects dogs of all ages. It produces scabs, which has given rise to word "scabies" as a common name for the disease. Other pets as well as people can get this form of mange.

Symptoms

The ailment generally starts on the bridge of the nose, around the eyes or at the base of the ears, although it may start elsewhere. Blisters form and a discharge from them dries and forms scabs which become branlike. There is intense itching with loss of hair. The skin becomes thickened and wrinkled.

Unless checked, the malady may cause digestive disturbances and other bodily ailments. Death may follow in a few months.

Sarcoptic mange closely resembles dry eczema and may be confused with demodectic (red) mange or ringworm. The

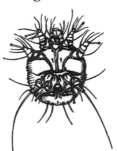

The sarcoptic mange mite, viewed from the under side. This mite is easy to kill.

mites are usually difficult to find—much more so than those of red mange. Persistent scraping of the skin with a sharp blade is necessary to dig them out. They cannot be identified without the aid of a microscope or perhaps a very strong magnifying glass.

Treatment

Sarcoptic mange responds well to proper treatment. Ointments containing flowers of sulfur are in common use and are available at pet supply dealers. An ointment can be made by mixing 1 part of flowers of sulfur with 8 parts of lard.

Ear Mange

EAR MANGE is caused by mites which look something like those that cause sarcoptic mange but are larger and have longer legs. They are white and slow-moving and can be seen without the aid of a microscope.

The mites live deep in the canal that leads from the outer ear to the eardrum. Here they burrow into the skin and feed on the tissue juices. The ear canal becomes filled with mites and modified wax. This causes intense itching. Affected dogs try to relieve this by scratching frantically and shaking their heads. Often an affected dog will hold its head to one side and when infection is severe will run in a circle or show other nervous signs.

Treatment

Treatment for ear mange consists in first carefully removing the accumulated wax and mites from the ear or ears. To avoid injury the dog should be tied or held firmly by an assistant. Wax can usually be removed with the help of eyebrow tweezers or the round end of a hairpin. Care should be used not to injure the eardrum which lies only a short distance in. The wax may also be removed by flushing out the ear with peroxide or a mixture of alcohol and ether. This mixture dissolves the wax.

After the wax is removed, the ear should be swabbed with any of several good medicines. Among these are a solution of glycerin and 1 percent phenol (carbolic acid); castor oil or olive oil containing 5 percent phenol; or a mixture of 1 part carbon tetrachloride and 3 parts castor oil. The treatment should be repeated daily until all traces of the mites are gone.

An ointment composed of 1 part, by measure, of derris powder containing 5 percent rotenone mixed with 10 parts of olive oil or vaseline is also effective. This usually kills the mites in one application but, to make sure, several weekly applications should be made.

How to Put an End to Ticks

THE HABITS of the various kinds of ticks are similar in many ways. They must all feed on blood in order to reproduce. The eggs are always deposited after the female has become engorged with blood and has dropped from the host.

The American dog tick is the most common one. It occurs nearly everywhere in the United States with the exception of two regions. These are the Rocky Mountain states where the Rocky Mountain fever tick holds sway, and in California and southern Oregon where the Pacific coast tick is common.

Other well-known ticks are the brown dog tick, the black-legged tick, the California black-legged tick, the Gulf coast tick and the lone star tick. All common ticks pass through four stages; the egg, seed tick or larva, nymph and adult.

Eggs of the American dog tick are laid on the ground in masses of 3,000 to 6,000. The eggs hatch into six-legged seed ticks which attach themselves to meadow mice or other small rodents. In a few days the ticks become filled with blood, drop to the ground and shed their skins. They emerge with eight legs and again attach themselves to small rodents to draw blood. This is the nymph stage. In three to ten days they drop to the ground, molt and emerge as adults.

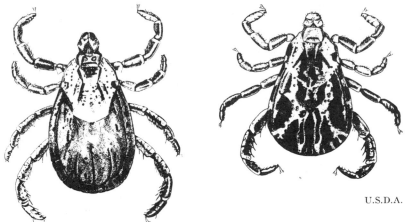

U.S.D.A.

Female and male ticks. Actually the male, on the right, should be proportionately somewhat smaller than shown. Both are of course greatly enlarged.

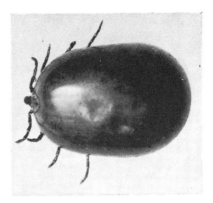

Here is a female dog tick that has filled herself with blood. A mixture of DDT and Lindane is used to kill ticks.

Both male and female adult ticks attach themselves to dogs where they engorge themselves with blood, and mate. Mating takes place while the females are feeding. In from five to 13 days, the females drop to the ground, lay their eggs and die. Their only food is the blood of mammals. Larvae and nymphs may live a year without feeding and adults may live two years.

The brown dog tick is particularly troublesome because it can live in houses or kennels with the dog as its only source of blood. In its several forms, it hides in furniture, in the folds of curtains, around baseboards or window casings. The adults, however, do not bite people. To get rid of the pests, it is of course necessary to destroy them in their hiding places on the premises as well as treating the dog.

Some ticks may transmit Rocky Mountain spotted fever and tularemia (rabbit fever) to human beings. However, these diseases do not occur in all localities where ticks are found and only a very small percentage of the ticks are infected where the diseases do occur.

Treatment

The most common drugs used for ticks are DDT and benzine hexachloride. A refined form of the latter drug is sold under the trade name of Lindane. It kills all kinds of lice and ticks. A spray containing 0.025 percent Lindane and 0.05 percent DDT is more satisfactory than Lindane alone.

Lindane will kill engorged forms of all common lice and ticks. DDT is relatively ineffective against engorged ticks but it remains on the animal longer and thus protects against reinfestation.

It's Easy to Kill Fleas and Lice

FLEAS NOT ONLY make life miserable for dogs but they may spread tapeworms, heartworms and under rare conditions bubonic plague.

The fleas that infest dogs are principally of four kinds: dog fleas, cat fleas, human fleas and sticktight fleas. The human flea may breed on dogs, cats and hogs as well as on people. Cat fleas prefer cats but will breed on dogs if no cats are around. Dog fleas prefer dogs but will nip palatable humans when no dogs are handy. Sticktight fleas also live on fowls and annoy humans.

The human flea is found mostly in the Mississippi Valley and in California. The sticktight flea is most common in southern states. Dog and cat fleas are found everywhere.

Female fleas produce large numbers of eggs which drop to the ground or floor or into the upholstery of furniture. These eggs hatch in a few days into maggotlike larvae, or worms, that are full-grown in two weeks or more, depending upon the temperature and the moisture present. These larvae spin cocoons about the size of wheat kernels.

After one week to several months, the fleas emerge, and if possible crawl up something so as to be about a foot above the ground. Here they wait for a dog or other host to pass, and jump to their new residence.

Sticktight fleas do not jump around like the other three

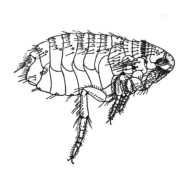
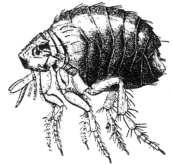

U.S.D.A.

At the left is the common dog flea and at the right, the sticktight flea.

kinds that infest dogs; they generally stay in one place. Often the ears of dogs become rimmed with hundreds of the pests.

Treatment

Any pet supply dealer sells a number of powders or lotions that will rid a dog of fleas. These usually contain rotenone, DDT, benzine hexachloride, Lindane, Toxaphene, derris root or cube root. Since fleas are continually picked up by dogs free to run at will, it is sometimes necessary to treat such animals every ten days or two weeks.

Eczema, or "Summer Itch"

ECZEMA, often called "summer itch," is one of the most common skin diseases of dogs. It is often mistaken for mange or ringworm. There are two kinds of eczema, a moist acute form, commonly called weeping eczema, and a dry chronic form. Both occur much more often in the summer than in the winter.

In the moist form, development of the disease is rapid. There is intense redness, marked itching, formation of blisters, loss of hair, and a glistening moist appearance of the skin. It occurs most often among long-haired dogs.

The dry or chronic type starts slowly. Symptoms are inflammation, eruptions of the skin, loss of hair, formation of crusts and scabs and intense itching. It occurs most often among coarse-haired dogs such as the wire-haired breeds.

Eczema develops most often around the base of the tail and along the back and shoulders. One moist form of the disease appears as a brownish discharge around the ear canal and between the toes.

The Cause of Eczema

There has been a wide difference of opinion on the cause of eczema. The malady has been attributed to food allergies, overfeeding, too much meat, too much starchy food, and vitamin or mineral deficiencies. But opinion has been changing in the past few years. The results of research and practical experience have shown that nearly all cases of eczema, where there is itching, and other symptoms as described above, are caused by infections of the skin.

It has been firmly established that one very common type of eczema is caused by the spores of a fungus, *Alternaria Tenuis,*

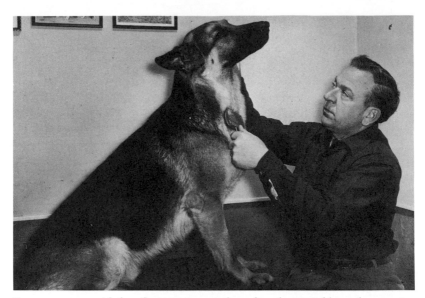

Someone once said that fleas were created so that dogs would not become too well satisfied with themselves. It's doubtful whether dogs concur in this belief.

which lives in dead grass and leaves. This fungus is microscopic in size. Like most fungi, it thrives in moist hot weather.

Treatment

Several kinds of fungicides are in use in treating eczema. One of these consists of zinc ointment to which has been added five to 20 grains of calomel for each ounce. Some of the newer patent dog medicines, especially those containing a drug called mercaptobenzothiazole, have been found highly effective. The drugs are of course applied to affected areas.

Since dogs can easily become infected again following treatment, it may be necessary to treat them several times during a summer.

Ringworm

RINGWORM is a contagious disease of the skin that some kinds of pets can get from one another and people can get from pets. It is caused by particular kinds of fungus.

In dogs, ringworm appears as small gray or brownish-yellow crusts that are usually round or oval in shape. Much of the hair falls out in the areas where ringworm occurs. The blotches usually appear on the face, head or legs but may occur elsewhere. Ringworm patches get larger as the disease progresses. The blotches disappear after awhile but new ones appear elsewhere. When the crusts are rubbed off to relieve itching, raw bleeding areas result. Sometimes there is little or no itching.

The disease is easily cured by medicines containing iodine, or salicylic acid or one of several other kinds of drugs. These are available in stores handling pet supplies.

Acne, or Pimples

ACNE IS AN infection of the hair follicles or glands of the skin. This causes pimples which break open and discharge pus. Scabs form over the openings in the skin while it is healing. The ailment often occurs under a dog's collar where dirt laden with germs is ground into the skin. Carbuncles, or boils, sometimes occur following acne.

Treatment

Treatment consists in breaking open pimples that are coming to a head, washing away the pus and treating the area with a non-irritating antiseptic such as Zonite or hydrogen peroxide. Ichthyol ointment rubbed firmly over the pimples before they have come to a head will sometimes kill the germs within and cause the pimples to disappear.

Death Knell for Lice

THREE kinds of lice infest dogs. Two of these are biting lice that feed on scales and other products of the skin. The third is a sucking louse that feeds on blood. Aside from their feeding habits, these lice resemble one another in most respects, though the biting lice have shorter heads and are usually more active.

Unlike fleas and ticks, lice may spend their entire lives on their hosts. The female attaches its eggs to hairs of the host. The eggs, called nits, hatch in five days and the emerging young reach adulthood in one to three weeks.

As is well known, lice irritate the skin, causing animals to bite and scratch themselves. Although lice will not breed when away from the host, they may live as long as five days off the host.

Treatment

A number of insecticides may be used to kill lice but most of them will not kill nits. For this reason, two applications are necessary, the second one twelve days after the first. The second application of insecticide kills the generation that hatches after the first application was made.

A few insecticides, developed in recent years, will kill both the lice and the nits. Among them are chlordane (0.5 percent solution) and toxaphene (0.75 percent solution). These, and similar chemicals, are contained in some of the patent medicines available at pet supply dealers.

Alopecia, or Loss of Hair

ALOPECIA is a fancy word for baldness or loss of hair. It may be natural—due to inheritance or old age, for example—or it may be caused by some disease such as distemper, diabetes or jaundice.

Dandruff

THE OUTER LAYER of skin of animals is constantly sloughing off. For reasons that are not known, this shedding of the outer skin, commonly known as dandruff, is more pronounced in some dogs than in others. About the only thing that can be done for dandruff is to brush the dog's coat frequently and bathe him often. In some cases, excessive dandruff is caused by lack of thyroid secretion.

Eye Diseases and Injuries

AILMENTS OF THE EYES are usually caused by one or the other of the following: general diseases which affect the eyes, such as distemper; local infections of the eye; mechanical injuries, also known as traumatic injuries. Eye ailments that are symptoms of other diseases are discussed under the various diseases in which they occur.

Conjunctivitis

Conjunctivitis is an inflammation of the edge of inner surface of the eyelids or the area around the eyeball. Treatment consists in flushing the eyes frequently with a warm 2-percent solution of boric acid, or placing in the eyes a drop or two of freshly prepared argyrol solution (5 to 10 percent), or a zinc sulfate solution (1 percent). The application of cold compresses two or three times a day will also help relieve the ailment.

Keratitis

Keratitis is an inflammation of the cornea, or covering of the front of the eyeball. It may be caused by wounds, such as cat scratches, foreign bodies or the spread of inflammation from other parts of the eye.

Symptoms are flow of tears, extreme sensitiveness to light and clouding of the cornea. This may vary from a milky-bluish transparent film to a yellowish-gray. Sometimes a film will cover the cornea without any apparent reason and will later disappear without ill effects. Treatment for keratitis is the same as for conjunctivitis.

Suppurative Keratitis

Suppurative keratitis is a disease in which ulcers appear on the eyes, varying in size from pin-point depressions to larger irregular areas containing pus. The healed ulcers sometimes leave scars that may impair the vision of a dog.

Treatment consists in bathing eyes in mild antiseptics such as 2-percent boric acid or by applying 1-percent yellow oxide

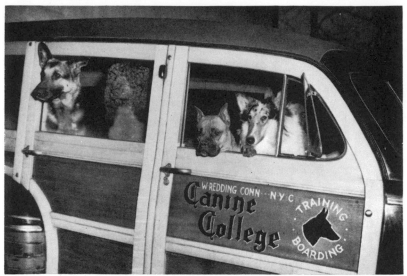

It's all right for these dapper college boys to look out of a station wagon window when the car is not moving, but not otherwise. Dogs stretching their heads from fast moving cars often suffer painful eye injuries.

or mercury ointment. Affected dogs should be kept from rubbing their eyes.

Pink Eye

Pink-eye is a malady in which the whole eye becomes inflamed. It is caused by microbes and is often highly contagious. The disease will usually disappear of its own accord but medicines will shorten its duration. The most effective treatment consists in applying ointments containing antibiotics such as penicillin or Bacitracin. Applications should be made in accordance with recommendations of the manufacturers.

Cataract

Cataract is a disease in which the lens of the eye becomes opaque. It is common among aged dogs but may sometimes occur among young ones as a result of injury or an attack of distemper. No medicinal treatment is known for the malady. It can sometimes be cured by an operation.

Glaucoma

Glaucoma is caused by increased pressure within the eye.

This enlarges and hardens the eyeball. It may occur in one or both eyes and causes some pain. Glaucoma usually develops slowly and does not occur until middle age. In most cases it is hereditary.

When only one eye is affected, it can be removed by surgery to bring relief but the operation is difficult.

What to Do About Running Fits

RUNNING FITS, often called fright disease, occurs in dogs of all breeds, at any age and at any time of the year. The ailment seems to occur more often in the South than in the North.

Before having an attack of running fits, a dog is usually restless, has a staring expression of the eyes and seems to be afraid of something. This is followed by running, barking and signs of excitement, together with other indications of great fear.

Attacks may last anywhere from a few minutes to half an hour or more. They may come on at intervals of a few days, weeks, or months. Attacks may occur only a few times or they may recur over a period of years. Dogs seldom die from the malady.

In mild attacks, dogs will hide following the period of excitement and reappear later seemingly with no ill effects. Champing of jaws, a heavy flow of saliva, spasms or convulsions may follow severe attacks. Some animals, especially hunting dogs, will occasionally yelp and run until exhausted.

The exact cause of running fits is not known. However, investigators at the Federal Bureau of Animal Industry have found that dogs that are allowed to run at will and which are on a diet consisting largely of meat seldom develop the disease.

Prevention and Treatment

From this it may be concluded that the disease can be largely prevented by giving dogs proper food and plenty of exercise. Some authorities believe that the tendency to running fits is inherited.

A dog with a running fit should be put in a dark room and kept free from annoyance. Recovery follows shortly.

Here's an Easy Way to Muzzle a Dog

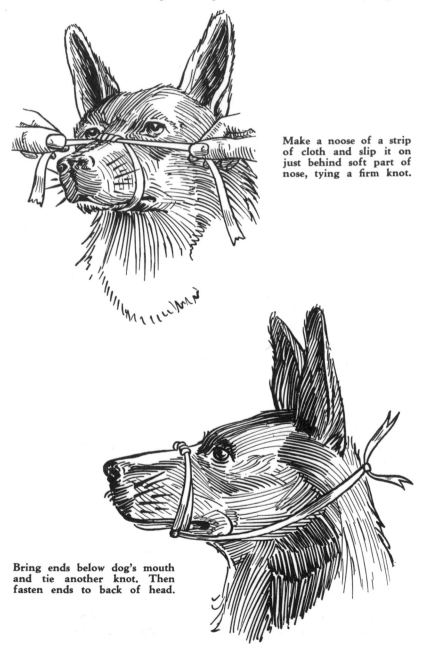

Make a noose of a strip of cloth and slip it on just behind soft part of nose, tying a firm knot.

Bring ends below dog's mouth and tie another knot. Then fasten ends to back of head.

Itchy Rectum

A DOG SOMETIMES sits down and propels himself across the ground or a floor by means of his front legs. Such a dog often indicates that he is in pain when he relieves himself. He may bite his rectum in an attempt to stop the itching.

Dog owners are apt to attribute such an itchy or sore rectum to the presence of worms. As a matter of fact, the symptoms generally indicate clogged or infected anal glands.

Dogs, skunks and a few other animals have two such glands, one on each side of the anus, or opening of the rectum. The anal glands give forth a grayish-brown substance with an offensive odor.

The purpose of these glands in the dog is not completely understood. It is known, however, that normally the glands are emptied quickly when a dog is terrified or even badly scared. In view of this, it is possible that the glands served to protect the dog's wild ancestors. It may be that the offensive odor made the dog undesirable as food for his enemies.

Treatment

In mild cases, the clogging of the openings of the anal glands can be relieved by pressing them between the thumb and forefinger. When an abscess has formed it may be necessary to gently cut open the glands and treat the infection with an antiseptic.

Sometimes infection of the anal glands causes eczema around the ears and eyes, spread to these parts when the affected dog licks and scratches himself. In such cases, the glands should be removed surgically — a comparatively simple operation. Following such an operation, penicillin is often used as an after-treatment to prevent infection.

Ear Canker

THERE are two kinds of ear canker: the external kind which affects the edges of the ear and the lobes, and the internal kind which involves the ear canal. The word canker, however, is loosely applied to many other ear infections.

External Canker

External ear canker most often affects dogs with long ears, such as hounds and setters. It is brought on by injuries, usually from bites, scratches and cuts, which later become infected. Fly bites, together with shaking of the head and scratching, often keep the wounded ears irritated and prevent healing. The usual symptoms are shaking of the head and pawing of the ears.

Treatment consists in cleaning the affected parts with soap and water to remove dried crusts; then applying antiseptic dusting powders daily.

Internal Canker

Internal ear canker is an infection of the ear canal, with inflammation, and a discharge that is usually brownish in color but may be yellowish. The discharge has an offensive odor and is usually of a waxy or cheesy nature though it may be a thick fluid. This discharge should not be confused with the ear wax caused by mites. The latter is drier, more crumbly and has less odor.

Treatment consists in cleaning the ear canal daily with swabs of cotton wound around a match or small stick and soaked in alcohol or ether. Swab carefully until ear is clean. Then apply a 2-percent solution of carbolic acid in sweet oil or glycerine. Or use one of the patent medicines specially compounded for treatment of the ailment.

Cases of long standing are sometimes hard to cure and require continued painstaking attention. When an internal canker persists, a veterinarian may find it necessary to open the ear canal at its lowest point, that is, below the ear. In this way any fluid present can be drained out and the infected part of the ear canal can be reached with antiseptics.

Dropsy, or Edema

WHEN FLUID collects in the body tissues or cavities, the condition is known as dropsy or edema. Such swollen tissues ooze fluid when the skin is broken. They are inelastic. When pressed with a finger, the tissues retain the imprint instead of springing back into place.

Dropsy is a symptom, not a disease. It may be caused by a number of body derangements but is most commonly due to bad kidneys, a weak heart, or a deranged liver.

Ascites

Ascites is a special kind of dropsy in which fluid collects principally in the abdomen. The swelling of the belly and usually of the limbs is easy to recognize. If water is given in only limited amounts, much of the swelling will disappear. The treatment must be drastic and most dog owners find it difficult to withstand the pleading of a thirsty pet. The water can be withdrawn from the abdomen by tapping but will again accumulate unless water is withheld.

Hydrothorax

Hydrothorax occurs when fluid accumulates in the chest cavity, other than in pleurisy. The principal symptom is shallow breathing. A dull thud is heard when the chest is tapped with the fingers, unlike the normal resonant sound. In severe cases, the lack of sufficient oxygen may cause the gums and tongue to become blue. Temperature is normal. The fluid can be drawn off by a veterinarian.

Pleurisy

PLEURISY is an inflammation of the coverings of the lungs usually accompanied with an accumulation of fluid in the chest cavity. The ailment often follows bronchitis and pneumonia. It may be caused by anything that permits certain microbes to enter the pleura, or covering of the lungs, such as broken ribs or foreign bodies. It is most likely to occur under cold damp conditions.

Pain is a principal symptom of pleurisy. Breathing is shallow and rapid, and produces an early crackling sound which later becomes grating, creaking or leathery. When fluid is present, a dull thud can be heard when affected areas are tapped with the fingers.

When there is a large accumulation of fluid, it should be drawn off. Pain should be relieved by giving patient aspirin. Dogs suffering from pleurisy should get the same care as recommended for pneumonia, described below.

Pneumonia

PNEUMONIA is an inflammation of the lungs caused by microbes. There are a number of different types of the disease but from the standpoint of symptoms they are nearly alike. Methods of treatment are similar.

The germs that cause pneumonia are nearly always present in the lungs of healthy animals but are held in check until an animal becomes weakened, or run down from another ailment. The malady often follows infectious diseases such as distemper. It may also be brought on by inhaling irritating substances such as dust and gases, sudden changes in temperature, exposure to rain and cold damp winds, and cold damp sleeping quarters.

Symptoms

Symptoms are shallow fast breathing, loss of appetite and fever of 104 to 105 degrees. Mucus may or may not flow from the nose. Usually a cough is present. Breathing causes a grating sound in the chest.

Treatment

The dog should be kept in a warm, well ventilated room free from drafts. If no warm place is available, then a sweater should be provided or the dog's chest should be loosely wrapped in warm material held in place with safety pins. Light appetizing foods should be provided, such as milk and beef extract. When the animal begins to get better, small amounts of meat and other nutritious foods should be given three or four times a day.

Medicinal treatment consists in injecting penicillin or giving aureomycin by mouth. If treatment is begun early in the course of the disease, the animal usually recovers in three or four days. When treatment is not begun until after the lungs are heavily involved, the blood does not circulate freely through the infected areas and the drugs do not serve their purpose.

Digestive Disturbances

DISORDERS of the digestion are common among dogs, most of them brought on by improper feeding. Vomiting, constipation and diarrhea are the most common symptoms although these disorders may also be caused by specific diseases.

Common Diarrhea and Constipation

Common diarrhea, the kind that is not brought on by internal parasites or infectious diseases, may sometimes be cleared up by adding small amounts of lime water, boiled rice and cheese to the diet. Bismuth subnitrate is also helpful, as is Kaopectate. The latter is available at drug stores. A teaspoonful should be given every two hours for a dog of medium weight. During this treatment, the dog should not be fed milk or eggs since these foods are slightly laxative. Other good remedies for diarrhea are available at pet supply dealers.

The common laxatives given dogs are of course the same as those used by human beings — mineral oil, castor oil, milk of magnesia, and so on.

Depraved Appetite

Dogs sometimes eat dirt and other indigestible materials. This may be due to lack of certain minerals or vitamins, to the presence of parasites, or to habit. Eating grass is also a habit of some dogs when they are thirsty or are suffering from a minor digestive disturbance.

Animals showing signs of depraved appetite should be kept in clean quarters, fed a balanced ration containing meat and milk, and given plenty of exercise.

Intestinal Obstructions

Dogs often swallow indigestible material which obstructs the intestine. Symptoms include loss of appetite, vomiting, bloating of the abdomen, and constipation. Mineral oil and enemas are given in treating this ailment, followed by a liquid diet.

Catarrhal Gastroenteritis

Gastroenteritis is an inflammation of the stomach and intestines. There are two kinds: catarrhal and hemorrhagic. According to "Keeping Livestock Healthy," a yearbook of the United States Department of Agriculture, both kinds are caused principally by improper feeding. Other causes are swallowing decomposed food, chemical poisons, internal parasites and infections by microbes.

Symptoms of catarrhal gastroenteritis are decrease in appetite, increased thirst, tenderness and pain in the region of the stomach. An affected dog may be uneasy, show stiffness in moving about and may vomit often. In severe cases, diarrhea develops. If not attended to, the ailment may become chronic.

In mild cases, the dog should be given no food for a day or two. Milk of magnesia, castor oil, or some other mild laxative should be given. In chronic cases in which there is frequent vomiting, the stomach should be irrigated with a weak solution of sodium bicarbonate.

Hemorrhagic Gastroenteritis

Hemorrhagic gastroenteritis is also called canine typhus and Stuttgart disease. Its symptoms include loss of appetite; persistent vomiting, at first of food only, later of blood and bile; weakness; an unpleasant peculiar odor of the breath; chocolate-colored discharge at the margins of the lips, and bloody diarrhea. As a rule there is no fever at any stage of the disease and there is no cough. Between 50 and 75 percent of affected animals die.

Dr. O. V. Brumley, noted veterinarian, Dean at Ohio State University, says the disease follows in the wake of dog shows and similar exhibitions. The nature of the disease, he says, indicates that it may be produced by some specific infection. The symptoms closely resemble those of blacktongue which, however, is definitely caused by a vitamin deficiency.

Treatment

Since water often induces vomiting, the affected dog should be given buttermilk instead. Food, consisting of raw fresh calf's liver, spleen, or liver extract, should be available but not forced upon the patient. When vomiting is heavy, the stomach should be irrigated with a 2-percent solution of sodium bicarbonate.

First Aid

WHEN A DOG is hit by an automobile, injuries often result that are not immediately apparent. There may be an internal hemorrhage, a bone dislocation or fracture, or an injury to the brain or a nerve.

For this reason an injured dog should be handled with utmost care, otherwise the injury may be made worse. Moreover, there is danger in handling an injured pet. When in a bewildered state, even the most friendly dog may become vicious and bite a person, not excluding his master.

Naturally, you want to call a veterinarian in case of severe injury, but often help is not at hand and immediate action is necessary to save a pet from further injury. When removing an injured dog from a street or highway, first make sure that he can't bite and then carry him carefully to a place of safety.

Profuse Bleeding

When blood oozes from a wound, it means that a vein has been cut. Such an injury is usually not serious. When blood flows from a wound in quick spurts, it means that an artery has been cut. The heavy loss of blood from such a wound may be serious.

Bleeding from a vein, or from an artery if it is not too severe, can usually be stopped by applying a pressure bandage directly over the wound. This is simply a wad of absorbent cotton or a wad of folded cloth held in place by a tightly wrapped bandage.

When bleeding from an artery is profuse, a tourniquet can often be used. This, however, should not be too tight and even when loosely applied, pressure should be released at intervals of about 20 minutes, otherwise gangrene may set in. A tourniquet is only for temporary use — to stop the flow of blood until it clots. It should of course be applied over an artery away from the wound and towards the heart. On a leg artery, for example, it should be applied above the wound.

Treating Bites and Cuts

Bites, cuts and abrasions of the skin are common among dogs. Don't bother about small scratches that a dog licks. Bites and larger cuts should first be washed with soap and water and then treated with a 2-percent solution of iodine or other good antiseptic. They should then be bandaged.

It sometimes happens that a dog injures a foot or some other part of his body and then keeps licking it so that it will not heal. If a bandage is applied, the dog promptly removes it. In such cases, an Elizabethan collar may be applied to advantage. Such a collar, named after those worn during the reign of the former queen of England, can be kept on a day or two while the wound is healing. (See page 75)

Shock

Shock is a condition associated with failure of the circulation of the blood. It may occur as a result of loss of blood, damage to tissues, a blow in a vital spot, or even emotional upsets. It

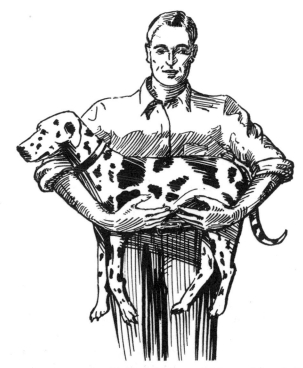

The utmost care should be used in carrying an injured dog.

varies from a condition resembling sleep to a severe form which may result in death.

The signs of shock vary with the cause and degree of shock. Breathing is rapid and shallow and the pulse rate is rapid.

The victim should be kept warm by covering him with a rug or other covering. A hot water bottle may also be used, provided care is taken not to burn the patient. To overcome shock, veterinarians often infuse glucose, dissolved in normal saline solution, into the veins. The latter solution is merely distilled water containing the same percentage of salt as the blood.

Burns and Scalds

For mild burns or scalds, cut away the hair and apply sterile vaseline, burn-ointment as sold in drug stores, olive oil or mineral oil. A 1-percent solution of picric acid, a freshly prepared 2½-to 5-percent tannic acid solution, or applications of saturated solutions of sodium bicarbonate are also widely used remedies. Strong freshly made tea may be used instead of tannic acid.

Bee and Wasp Stings

Dogs have a habit of snapping at bees and wasps, a practice that is not always to their advantage. To relieve the discomfort of a sting, first remove stingers, then apply weak ammonia water or a paste of baking soda and water.

Snake Bite

A poisonous snake bite is rapidly followed by severe pain and swelling and calls for quick action. If professional help is not immediately available, you'll have to do the best you can.

Two things should be accomplished by treating a snake bite: First, expel as much poison as possible from the wound, second, keep the poison that remains, from spreading to other parts of the body.

With the point of a knife or a razor blade — preferably after passing it through the flame of a match—make a cross cut in the shape of the letter X over each fang mark. These cuts should be from 1/8 to ¼ inch deep. Remember that the fangs penetrate at an angle so it is best to have top and bottom crosses join each other. Squeeze out the blood. If a suction device is at hand, use it to draw blood from the wound. Drop

So Dogs Will Let Their Wounds Alone

The "Elizabethan collar" at the right is made of corrugated paper, reinforced with adhesive tape.

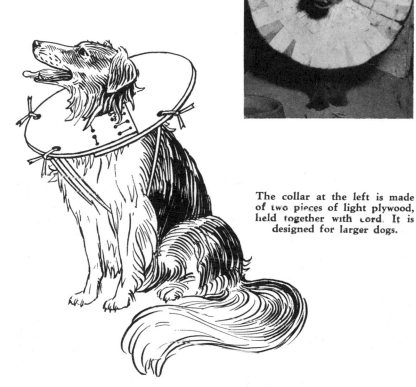

The collar at the left is made of two pieces of light plywood, held together with cord. It is designed for larger dogs.

The head funnel at the right may be made of heavy cardboard or plastic. It prevents a dog from scratching a sore head or ears.

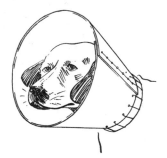

potassium permanganate (from a drug store) into the wound. Apply a tourniquet as described above under "profuse bleeding."

Frostbite

If the victim of frostbite cannot immediately be brought to warm shelter, warm the frozen part by covering it with the hand and then apply a piece of old blanket or other material. This will restore circulation.

Frostbitten areas should be thawed out gradually. Do not rub a frozen area, especially not with snow or ice. Frozen tissues are easily bruised or torn and if this occurs, gangrene may result.

Car Sickness

Dogs often get car sick, especially those with a nervous disposition. Drooling and vomiting are the symptoms.

The ailment can often be prevented by withholding food and water for an hour before starting on a journey, also by giving

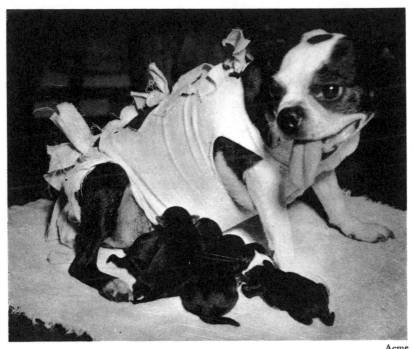

Acme

Now and then dogs, too, need emergency operations. This bitch is nursing her litter following a Caesarian.

the dog an opportunity to empty his bowels and bladder. Tablets containing sodium bromide are sometimes given a dog before starting on a journey to prevent vomiting. These are obtainable at drug stores. The medicine should be given as prescribed for human beings, but in proportion to the weight of the dog as compared with that of a person. Do not overdose.

Removing Objects from Throat

When a dog is choking from a foreign object caught in the throat, press the thumb and forefinger of one hand into cheeks of the animal, thus forcing him to open his mouth wide. Then try to reach the object with the fingers. If forceps are not at hand, long-nose plyers may serve to grasp a bone or other object that is stuck below the point where it can be reached with the fingers.

Bloat

Sometimes a dog will gorge himself with a food that forms gas so rapidly that the gas cannot escape fast enough. The stomach then becomes bloated. If a severe case of bloat is not relieved the animal will die.

If you cannot get a veterinarian promptly when bloat occurs, first try to release the gas by running a rubber tube gently into the animal's stomach by way of the throat. If this doesn't help, then a more drastic method should be used. To release the gas, the stomach must be punctured from the outside.

Veterinarians puncture a stomach by means of a trocar, a sharp-pointed instrument encased in a sheath called a cannula. The trocar is stuck through the affected dog's right side just behind the ribs. The trocar is then withdrawn and the cannula remains — a tube with an inner diameter a little larger than that of a bean blower. Through this tube, the gas escapes and the bloat subsides.

If you do not have a trocar, a piece of metal tubing can be used after sharpening the end for easier penetration. If neither are at hand, use the long blade of a knife. This is better than letting the dog die. If a tube becomes clogged with food, remove the obstacle with a piece of wire.

Coccidiosis

COCCIDIOSIS, pronounced "cock-siddy-o-sis," is caused by parasites that live in the small intestines. These parasites multiply and later become egglike in form, when they are known as oocysts, which pass out of the intestines into the stool. A few days later they are infective, that is, they will infect other dogs if they find their way into a dog's intestines.

Symptoms
Mild cases of coccidiosis are without observable symptoms. With more severe infections, symptoms are diarrhea, which may be bloody, gas, small appetite, coughing, and sometimes a rise in temperature to about 103 degrees. Death may result with heavy infections among young or very weak animals.

Positive diagnosis is made by finding the oocysts in the stools of animals by means of a microscope.

The infection runs a regular course and then dies out. Thereafter an infected animal is immune to that particular type of coccidiosis although it may get another type.

Treatment
A number of treatments are in use. Among them are the sulfa drugs, bone phosphate and kaolin. Since the disease is usually not serious and has a tendency to die out after an animal is about six months old, there is often doubt as to whether a treatment is worth bothering with.

Salmon Poisoning

SALMON POISONING is caused by eating salmon infested with a certain kind of fluke. The malady occurs in California, Oregon, Washington and Southwestern Canada. This fluke is a tiny, flattened worm, barely visible to the unaided eye.

When salmon infected with flukes are eaten by dogs, the parasites are released in the small intestines. Here they develop into mature flukes in five to ten days. Research men have proved, however, that the disease is caused by a microbe associated with the flukes and not by the flukes themselves.

The onset of salmon disease is sudden. Temperature goes to between 105 and 107 degrees. The animal refuses to eat, is extremely thirsty, seems depressed and has a discharge from its eyes. The face is often swollen which makes the eyes appear sunken.

In 24 to 48 hours the temperature drops and diarrhea sets in. The stool is at first tinged with blood and later consists almost entirely of blood. The animal becomes weak and thin. In about a week, its temperature drops below normal. Death usually follows in a few days.

Between 50 and 90 percent of untreated animals die. Those that survive are thereafter immune to the disease.

Prevention and Treatment

The disease can be prevented by not feeding dogs with uncooked fish of the salmon family. Other kinds of uncooked fish should also be avoided since they often harbor other flukes that cause disease. Salmon disease has been successfully treated with certain sulfa drugs and with penicillin.

Piroplasmosis

PIROPLASMOSIS is transmitted from dog to dog by ticks, especially by the brown dog tick. The disease may occur wherever there are ticks but is practically unknown in many areas. It occurs most often in southern states, particularly in Florida.

In the acute form of the disease, outward symptoms resemble those of distemper. Temperature rises, breathing becomes rapid, pulse rate increases. There is increased thirst, loss of appetite, and reddening of the visible mucous membranes—the gums, lips and around the eyes. Urine usually becomes reddish brown. Jaundice is present in about half the cases. Affected animals frequently die.

In the chronic form, fever occurs at first and in rare instances appears intermittently. Affected dogs are listless, there is loss of weight and diminished appetite. Mucous membranes are pale instead of red. Jaundice is usually absent though it may appear in the later stages of the disease.

Piroplasmosis is caused by a microbe called *Piroplasma canis* which is so small that it lives inside of the red blood cells. Laboratory diagnosis consists in microscopic examination of the red blood corpuscles. Since in chronic cases, the *Piroplasma* are often hard to find, where valuable dogs are involved, blood from sick animals is sometimes injected into susceptible puppies. The blood of the puppies will contain the microbes in about four to seven days. Both the older dogs and the puppies are then treated for the disease.

Treatment
Treatment consists in hypodermic injection of a 0.5 percent ($\frac{1}{2}$ of 1%) solution of acapron. The dose is $\frac{1}{4}$ cc for each 10 pounds of body weight. One injection effects a cure in 90 percent of the cases. Symptoms disappear in 24 hours. In case of relapse, a second injection may be given. An overdose of the drug may kill the dog. Acapron should be given only as a hypodermic injection. It sometimes has side effects consisting of restlessness, tremors and flow of saliva but these will pass away.

Canine Leptospirosis

LEPTOSPIROSIS is an infectious disease that affects all breeds of dogs. It is spread largely by rats but also spreads from dog to dog. The microbes are contained in the urine of the infected animals. The disease spreads rapidly and is often fatal. Humans may also contract the malady, in which case it is known as Weil's disease or infectious jaundice.

Symptoms
The disease is difficult to diagnose in its early stages because in the beginning, symptoms resemble those of distemper, hepatitis and nephritis.

There are two types of leptospirosis, caused by different microbes, the *canicola* and the *ictero-hemorrhagic* types. They have some symptoms in common. The latter type is the more severe.

Common symptoms are dullness, loss of weight, stiffness in the hindquarters, loose stools and a temperature of 103.5 to 106 F. Another sign which is nearly always present is congestion of the tiny arteries in the whites of the eyes, often giving them a coppery tinge. In the latter course of the disease the temperature drops to normal or below normal. Slight pressure over the kidneys is painful to an affected dog.

In the *canicola* type of the malady, the urine may contain blood or may be orange or chocolate brown in color.

The principal symptom of the ictero-hemorrhagic type of leptospirosis is jaundice. The whites of the eyes, the inside of the mouth and finally the skin become more and more yellow as the disease progresses.

Treatment and Prevention

By the time jaundice is noticed so much damage has usually been done to the liver and kidneys that recovery is impossible.

In young dogs and vigorous older animals, the disease can be cured in its early stages by giving large doses of penicillin. A high blood level of the drug should be kept for at least five days, otherwise a relapse usually occurs. The recommended dosage is 450,000 to 600,000 units a day for the first two days, followed by 300,000 units for the remainder of the period.

To prevent occurrences of the leptospirosis, premises should be rid of rats. It has been estimated that between 30 and 50 percent of all rats are carriers of the disease.

Histoplasmosis

HISTOPLASMOSIS is a comparatively rare disease caused by a fungus called *Histoplasma capsulatum*. It affects dogs, humans, mice, rats, rabbits and horses. It is not known how the malady is spread.

Symptoms

The disease, in dogs, usually occurs in one of two forms, chronic or benign. Signs most often observed in the chronic form are dysentery, cough, loss of appetite and weight and vomiting. These symptoms are followed by inflammation of the skin, irregular fever, labored breathing, anemia, arthritis and jaundice.

The cough persists and no way has been found to relieve it. When dysentery occurs. the stool contains mucus and is sometimes blood-streaked. This form of histoplasmosis is always fatal.

With the benign form of the disease, a dog may live for

years without showing any outward symptoms. An accurate skin test used by veterinarians and laboratory men shows whether or not the disease is present. Post mortem examinations reveal derangements of the liver, spleen and other internal organs.

No cure for the disease has been found.

Trichinosis

TRICHINOSIS is caused by small roundworms that become imbedded in the muscles. The disease occurs in many meat-eating animals including dogs.

It is spread principally by eating raw or undercooked pork. Dogs, however, may get the disease by eating the flesh of certain other meat-eating animals such as rats and mice which in turn have eaten infected pork. Hunting dogs sometimes become infected from eating the flesh of wild animals that are meat eaters.

In mild cases of trichinosis, symptoms are not noticeable. In severe cases symptoms are fever and muscular pain. The disease is difficult to diagnose. The worms, called *Trichinae,* may be found by examining a thin layer of infected meat under a microscope, but even this method is not completely dependable.

There is no effective treatment for the disease. Prevention consists in not permitting the dogs to eat undercooked pork or other flesh that may be infected.

Abnormal Growths and Swellings

THE COMMON forms of abnormal growths on dogs are abscesses, cysts, tumors, warts, hernias and enlargements of some of the glands that lie near the surface of the body.

Abscess

An abscess is an enlargement filled with pus, commonly called a boil. It may appear anywhere on the body and often occurs following a scratch, bite or other puncture of the skin that is not kept clean and as a result becomes infected.

An abscess should not be squeezed or opened until it is "ripe," that is, until it looks as though it were almost ready to break open of its own accord. If the abscess is tampered with before a pocket, or sac, has been formed around the pus, the infection may get into the blood stream with serious results. Hot applications will help draw an abscess to a head.

Sometimes an abscess seems to ripen but will not come to a head. In such cases it should be lanced—cut open with a sharp knife or razor blade. Use extreme care so as to cut only through the outer covering of the abscess. If you cut all the way through the pus sac, microbes may enter the blood and the animal may die.

After the pus has been removed from an abscess, the wound should be treated with a good antiseptic such as tincture of iodine or Zonite. The wound should be kept open so that it does not heal over, but heals from the inside outward. (See page 87)

Care must be taken not to confuse a hernia, cyst or other growth with an abscess.

Hematoma, a Type of Cyst

A cyst is an enlargement that looks like a tumor but is filled with a fluid or a semifluid substance. There are a number of different kinds of cysts, but the most common among dogs is a blood cyst, or hemotoma, of the ear. This is sometimes caused by an accidental injury or by scratching but perhaps more often by frequent shaking of the ear flap, particularly against collar hardware.

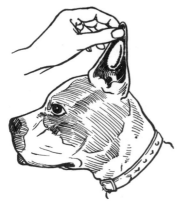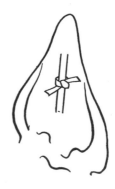

Ear hematomas like the one at the left may be drained by making two incisions as shown at the right. The piece of gauze keeps the wound open until it has drained.

Ear hematomas usually appear on the inside of the ear flaps. They consist of pockets filled with blood and lie between the layers of skin. Small hematomas, commonly called blood blisters, usually disappear of their own accord. Large ones should be cut open and drained.

There are several ways to operate on a hematoma. In all of them, the object is to remove all of the contents of the swelling. To do this it is necessary to keep the wound from healing until it has drained. If the blood is not drained off, it will clot. If the clot remains, it will later shrink and the ear will be deformed.

Before treatment, the animal should be put under an anesthetic. This may be either a general or local.

After shaving off the hair, make two incisions as shown in the drawing on this page. Clean out blood clots and stringy material. Insert a sterile piece of gauze underneath the strip of skin as shown. The gauze should be moved back and forth once a day to reopen the wound so it can be drained properly. Flush out with a mild antiseptic solution.

After the outer flaps of skin start to adhere to the surface underneath the gauze should be removed. The strip of skin will soon grow back into place.

Tumors

Tumors are abnormal growths of tissue. There are two general types—malignant tumors which develop rapidly and

84

may spread to other parts of the body, and benign tumors which grow slowly and are confined to one part of the body.

A malignant tumor is commonly called a cancer. Unless removed, malignant tumors usually cause death. Benign tumors often grow to a large size and cause discomfort but an animal may live for years with such a growth, particularly if it is on the outside of the body. A malignant tumor has the tendency to come back if removed whereas a nonmalignant, or benign tumor will usually not recur if cut off.

The most common and most dangerous malignant tumor is known as a carcinoma. It occurs almost exclusively among adult dogs, particularly older ones. It commonly occurs in the throat or in mammary gland although it may occur elsewhere. This cancer is hard to the touch and has well-defined edges. Loss of weight usually accompanies a malignant cancer.

When a cancer occurs in the region of the mouth or throat, it is painful for a dog to chew or swallow. After attempting to eat, such an animal will often acquire a haggard look and will droop its head in a dejected and pathetic manner. Often the first signs are an angry looking growth on the gums or a sore near a tonsil. The animal shows pain when these spots are touched.

It is usually difficult if not impossible to tell one kind of

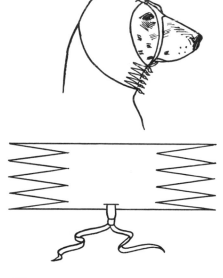

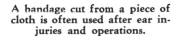

A bandage cut from a piece of cloth is often used after ear injuries and operations.

tumor from another without a microscopic examination of the tissue. Tumors should be removed as soon as possible to prevent later suffering.

Mumps

Mumps is an enlargement of the salivary glands, caused by infection or injury. The glands affected lie below the ears and are called the parotid glands. The disease is technically known as parotitis.

The head and neck may become enlarged. An affected dog has difficulty in swallowing, has fever, and abscesses may form in one or both of the glands. The saliva is often thick and ropy.

Mumps can be cured with some of the antibiotics and sulfa drugs. The abscesses are often opened in severe cases. Incisions are made at the bottom of the swellings so that the pus drains out more easily.

Goiter

Goiter is an enlargement of the thyroid gland and appears as a swelling at both sides of the lower part of the windpipe. There is no pain and the swelling is not overly warm. In size it may be anywhere between that of a walnut and an apple. A goiter often makes breathing difficult.

The common method of treatment consists in applying tincture of iodine to the swelling every day for four or five days. Good results have been obtained by giving thyroid extract. Operations to cure goiter are extremely dangerous.

Hodgkin's Disease

Hodgkin's disease is marked by swelling of the lymphatic glands, including enlargement of the spleen. The cause of the malady is not known.

The swelling of the lymph nodes can be felt. Other symptoms are rapid breathing, anemia and dropsy, or puffy swelling of the abdomen.

The course of the disease is rapid. Veterinarians sometimes prescribe arsenic compounds to relieve the ailment, especially the one known as sodium cacodylate.

Warts

There are two kinds of warts: hard and soft. Hard warts are round and smooth and occur especially on the eyelids,

An Abscess Needs Careful Treatment

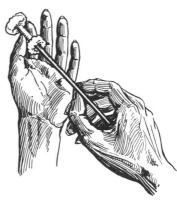

Right: Twist some cotton over the end of a round stick. Dip the cotton in a good antiseptic solution.

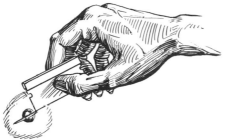

Left: Cut through the skin covering the abscess with a sharp knife or razor blade.

Right: Gently squeeze out the pus and remove it with a piece of cotton.

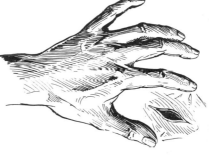

Left: Insert the cotton at the end of the stick into the wound. Cut it off below the end of the stick, as shown. Hold the cotton plug in place with a piece of adhesive tape and let the wound heal from the inside outward.

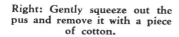

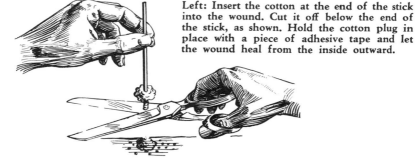

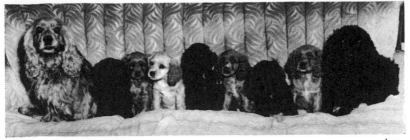

The tendency among dogs to have warts and other growths is largely inherited.

backs and necks of old dogs. Soft warts are flat, rough and cauliflowerlike in appearance. They occur principally in the mouths and on the genital organs of young dogs.

Warts seldom do any harm although they may interfere with eating and cause excessive flow of saliva when in the mouth in large numbers. The tendency among dogs to have warts is largely inherited.

Many treatments are in use for removing warts, including surgery. The application of carbon dioxide snow, glacial acetic acid, salicylic acid ointment, and oil of thuja are some of the common medicinal remedies. Soft warts sometimes disappear without treatment.

Rupture, or Hernia

A RUPTURE, or hernia, is an enlargement, usually of the wall of the abdomen, caused by an opening which permits the intestines or other internal organs to protrude. Most hernias do not break through the skin. Among dogs, the tendency to have hernias is largely inherited.

There are several kinds of hernias and they occur with varying degrees of severity. Small ones may usually be disregarded without fear of serious consequences.

Care should be taken not to confuse a hernia with various growths that may appear on the abdomen. In most cases a hernia will disappear when an affected dog is laid on his back whereas other growths will not.

Umbilical Hernia

The most common hernia among dogs is the kind where the intestines protrude at the navel, called an umbilical hernia. A puppy is often born with such a hernia but it usually disappears as the animal grows older. If not, an operation may be necessary.

Either a local or general anesthetic may be used in operating. The protruding hernia should be pushed back into the abdomen and any adhesions should be carefully separated. The sac formed by the distended inner lining of the body cavity should be dissected (cut) out, and the opening should be sutured (stitched) with catgut.

The edges of the muscles surrounding the wound should then be scraped so they will grow together more easily following the operation. The skin should be sutured with silk and the wound dusted with penicillin.

To keep the dog from tearing out the stitches and keep the wound clean, the abdomen should be covered with a thin cloth jacket until the wound has healed. In addition, an "Elizabethan collar" may be used, as shown on page 75.

Scrotal and Inguinal Hernias

When the intestines break through the ring in the abdomen

through which the spermatic cord passes to the testicles, the result is what is called a scrotal hernia. A loop of the intestines becomes imprisoned in the scrotum, or "bag." In severe cases, even the bladder may descend into the scrotum. The operation to reduce (cure) this type of hernia is difficult, particularly since, in suturing, care must be taken not to interfere with the spermatic cord.

An inguinal hernia is an incomplete scrotal hernia. In this case a portion of the bowel passes through the internal inguinal ring (the opening into the scrotum) but does not descend into the scrotum. Inguinal hernia appears as an enlargement at one side of the penis.

Inguinal hernia in the bitch is more common than in the male. It appears as an enlargement just back of the inguinal mammae, the hindmost of the teats. The enlargement may be a small rounded mass or large enough to reach the ground.

Other Kinds

A diaphragmatic hernia occurs commonly following an accident. In such cases the liver, intestines or other internal organs pass through a rent in the diaphragm that separates the abdominal from the chest cavity.

Perineal hernia is an ailment of the male dog which generally does not occur until the animal has passed middle age. It results from an enlarged prostate gland which causes an animal to feel that there is a stool in the bowel when actually there is not. In trying to pass this stool, the dog strains himself and weakens the muscles and other tissues surrounding the anus, the opening to the rectum. Eventually the inner membrane is torn and the bowels and other organs of the pelvis protrude, making a bulge in the animal's rear.

How to Dock Tails

WE HAVE BECOME so accustomed to seeing some breeds of dogs with their tails docked that such dogs just don't look right with long tails. Most terrier types of dogs look sort of ridiculous with long tails.

Sometimes friendly dogs wag their tails almost constantly and with such vigor that they are continually injuring their tails. Docking then becomes necessary to protect these animals. Open wounds from tail wagging often become infected.

In docking a dog, the amount of tail to cut off varies with the breed of dog and with the fashion at the time. The easiest way to determine how long the stump should be is to observe other fine dogs of the same breed. The tendency among amateurs is to cut tails too short. In spaniels, the length of the stump is not so important. Their long hair covers the stump so that its actual length is not particularly noticeable. On the other hand, to dock a Doberman Pinscher too long or a wire-haired terrier too short may detract somewhat from the appearance of these animals.

The best time to dock tails is when the animals are pups— under a week old and preferably under 48 hours old. At this early age, puppies suffer very little pain so no anesthetic is necessary. Dogs over six months should be given an anesthetic before their tails are docked. Unless absolutely necessary such dogs should not be docked at all.

Before docking a tail, clip the hair at the place where the cutting is to be done and treat the area with an antiseptic such as tincture of iodine or Zonite. Cutting may be done with a pair of bone shears, pruning shears or a sharp knife. Before cutting, the skin of the tail should be pulled towards the body. This is done so that the skin will go back in place and cover the stub after the operation is completed.

The tail stubs of puppies should not be bandaged since this is not necessary and moreover the dam will usually remove a bandage anyway. Some veterinarians cauterize the stump by applying a hot iron lightly to the open wound. This sears the blood vessels and prevents bleeding. In most cases bleeding stops of its own accord and the wound heals without any trouble. A dam should be prevented from licking the wounds of her puppies, otherwise the wounds will not heal. If necessary puppies should be taken away from the dam except when nursing.

When it is necessary to dock older dogs, the method is the same as with young ones, except the animal should be given an anesthetic and the stump of the tail should be wrapped in gauze or otherwise protected from dirt while it is healing.

Ear Cropping

EAR CROPPING is illegal in Great Britain. Many people think it should be made illegal in America. However, since public demand makes the operation common practice in the United States, a brief discussion of it rightfully belongs in this book.

In Great Danes, Doberman Pinschers and Boxers the best time to crop ears is at the age of 10 to 12 weeks. In Bull Terriers, Boston Terriers, Toy Manchesters and other small breeds it is better to wait until dogs are between four and six months old.

When having their ears cropped, dogs should always be good

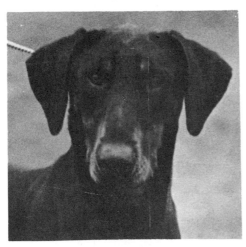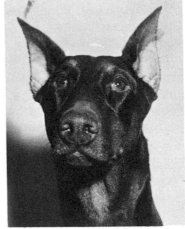

To dog fanciers, some breeds of dogs don't look natural unless their ears have been cropped.

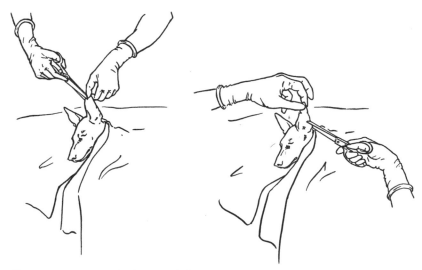

Some operators notch the ears before cutting. This is done to guide them in removing the same amount from each ear.

surgical risks. They should be free from parasites and in good physical condition.

Before starting to operate, clip the hair from the ears, both inside and outside and wash the ears and the upper part of the head with soap and water. Thoroughly dry all washed areas. Treat the ears with 70 percent alcohol or some other suitable antiseptic. Plug the ears with cotton.

An operator can do his best work if the patient is under complete anesthesia. This practice is of course also the most humane.

As with tail docking, the style of trim should conform to the style that prevails among dogs of the particular breed being operated on. Plan the work in advance. Never whittle on an ear to attain a certain shape.

When ready to operate, drape the ears over the head and nick them top and bottom in accordance with the desired contour. This helps to equalize the amount to be trimmed from each ear.

Right-handed operators tend to cut off more of the right ear than the left. You can guard against this to a large extent by using the cut-off portion of one ear as a pattern. Simply lay the cut-off piece on the draping cloth in an inverted position near the ear to be trimmed and follow the outline.

To stop bleeding, veterinarians compress the arteries with forceps (pincers) that can be tightened into place. Sometimes arteries are ligated (a thread tied around them) to stop the flow of blood.

Suturing (sewing) can be done best with size 00 or 000 catgut. Stitches should be made so that the skin is flush with the margin of the cartilage but does not extend beyond it. Begin stitches at the base of the ears. Using a continuous stitch, pass the needle through both the skin and the cartilage. Not more than two-thirds to three-quarters of the ear need be sutured.

After the operation, wipe the blood from the wounds and apply 2-percent tincture of iodine, penicillin or some other good germicide to the wounds. Apply sterile bandages, folding the ears over the top of the head. With small dogs these may be removed in 48 hours without further attention. With large dogs, frames to hold the ears upright are usually fixed to the ears with adhesive tape and kept there for four days.

How to Give an Anesthetic

MOST OF THE ANESTHETICS used by veterinarians can be obtained only on prescription. Two that can be bought freely by laymen are chloroform and ether.

The use of chloroform is dangerous because a dog, if given a small overdose, may die virtually without warning. With ether, on the other hand, there are signs of an overdose before the danger point is reached. Ether, however, has one disadvantage: it is highly explosive. A lighted match or the pilot light on a gas stove may explode the fumes.

Before giving ether, a dog should be securely tied. A kitchen table or a work bench will serve as an operating table. The eyes of the animal should be protected against the ether by wrapping a cloth around the face and eyes.

Ether may be given by saturating a folded towel with it and holding the towel close to the dog's nose. Another way to give it consists in putting cotton in a tin can with holes punched in the cover and saturating the cotton with ether before putting the cover on. The can should be held so that the dog inhales the fumes.

Four stages of ether anesthesia are generally recognized by veterinarians. In the first stage, which lasts one or two minutes, the animal is excited and delirious. Breathing becomes rapid and there is an increased flow of saliva.

As more ether is taken into the lungs, the dog enters the second stage. Breathing becomes more moderate and more regular and the body becomes relaxed. Painless operations may be performed in this stage but the animal is still sensitive to pain.

In the third stage of anesthesia, breathing becomes deep, regular and quiet. The animal is completely relaxed and insensitive to pain. The pupils of the eyes are somewhat enlarged. This is the stage in which surgery should be performed.

The fourth stage is the recovery stage. Within a few minutes after ether is withdrawn, the patient begins to regain consciousness. At first, breathing is intermittent and weak but normal breathing soon follows.

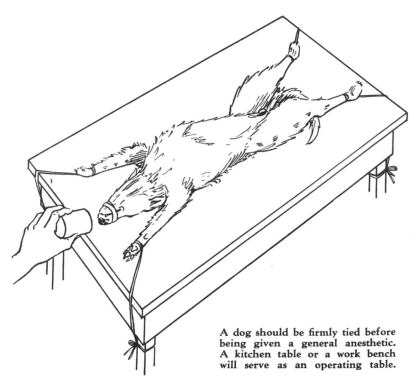

A dog should be firmly tied before being given a general anesthetic. A kitchen table or a work bench will serve as an operating table.

An overdose of ether paralyzes the nerves that control breathing. But the nature of the breathing forewarns the operator of impending paralysis. The operator or an assistant, should constantly watch the respiration of the patient.

If breathing is shallow, it indicates either that the anesthetic has not as yet produced its full effect, or that the animal is getting an overdose. If full anesthesia has not been obtained, the pupils will become smaller when a flashlight is shone on them. If breathing is shallow and there is no response to light, the ether should be withdrawn at once. Except at the beginning of anesthesia, irregular breathing is also a danger signal and calls for immediate withdrawal of ether.

If an animal stops breathing, or if there is danger of it, start artificial respiration at once. This is done by laying the dog on his side and pushing his ribs in with the flat of the hand. Release quickly and repeat pressure at intervals of about once every two seconds.

Medicines——Their Use and Abuse

THE LAW requires that a medicine sold to the public without a prescription must be properly labeled. Among other things, the label must tell exactly what drugs the medicine contains and how the medicine should be used.

Always follow directions of the manufacturers. If you use a larger dose than recommended, you may injure your dog or even kill him; if you use a smaller dose, the medicine may not do any good.

Most drugs are specific in their action, that is, they serve to relieve a definite ailment and are of no use in treating any other disease. There is no such thing as a "cure-all" medicine. The random use of so-called tonics serves no useful purpose.

Medicines Are Usually Mixtures

Drugs are seldom given in their pure form. They are nearly always mixed with water, alcohol, oil, or some other so-called vehicle. This is done principally to make it easier to give the medicine to the patient and to insure greater accuracy in the size of the dose. Medicines to be given by mouth generally contain some harmless substance that makes them taste better.

The size of a dose of medicine for a dog should usually vary in accordance with his weight. For example, a dog weighing 100 pounds should be given twice as large a dose as one weighing 50 pounds. With some drugs, however, a large dog should not be given quite so large a dose proportionately as a small dog.

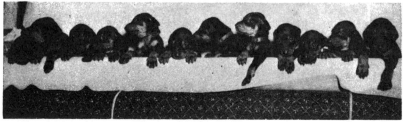

International

In general, the size of a dose of medicine should vary in accordance with a dog's weight. Always follow directions of manufacturers.

Many drugs cannot be sold to the public without a prescription. Some of these, however, may be included in patent medicines, provided that the manufacturers of the medicines abide by certain provisions of the law.

Before treating a dog it is of course necessary to find out what ails him. If he can be cured by means of a medicine, get the kind required.

Medicines are given most often in the form of liquids, pills tablets or powders, although injections are also quite common.

How to Give a Liquid Medicine

In giving a dog a liquid medicine, do not open the mouth. Instead, pull out the lower lip at the corner of the mouth and pour the medicine in with a spoon or bottle. Should the dog hold the medicine in his mouth, he can be made to swallow it by opening the mouth slightly.

The head should be held very slightly upward. If held too high, the medicine may enter the windpipe instead of the pass-

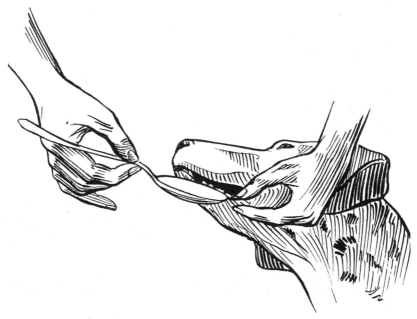

Liquid medicines may be given either from a spoon or from a bottle.

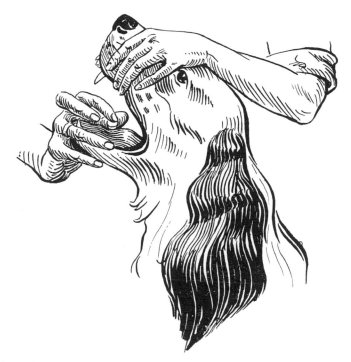

To give a dog a pill, hold the upper jaw with the left hand and rest the right hand on the lower jaw, placing the pill quite far back on the tongue.

age to the stomach and cause choking. In case of a vicious animal, the medicine can still be given by this method, even though the dog's mouth is held shut with a tape.

Pills, Tablets and Powders

To give a dog a pill or tablet, open his mouth by placing your left thumb on the roof of the mouth behind the canine tooth. Pressure with the thumb will make nearly all dogs open their mouths and they seem unable to close them until the pressure is released. With the right hand, place the pill or tablet far back on the tongue, then take out your thumb and close the mouth. The medicine will be swallowed.

Powders are given in the same manner as pills except that powders are dropped on the back of the tongue from the papers in which they are wrapped.

Bone Fractures

THERE ARE A NUMBER of different kinds of fractures, named in accordance with the manner in which the bone is injured.

A simple fracture is one where there is a clean break and there is little if any injury to the surrounding flesh.

A compound fracture is one in which the bone is broken through the skin.

A comminuted fracture is one in which the bone is broken into several fragments.

A greenstick fracture is one that occurs in young dogs and puppies before their bones have hardened. The bone is really not broken in two but is cracked and usually bent out of shape.

Symptoms of a Fracture

The symptoms of a fracture are pain; loss of the use of the broken bone; unnatural movability, such as a dangling leg, and swelling of the surrounding area. Except in case of a greenstick fracture, there is also a grating sound or a feeling of grating bones when a broken bone is manipulated. This is particularly noticeable in case of a broken limb where the bone is broken into two parts. The muscles attached to such a limb pull the parts in such a way that they overlap.

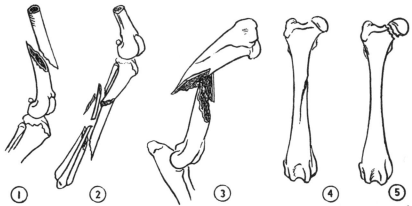

1—Simple oblique fracture (Bones do not penetrate skin). 2—Comminuted fracture of radius and ulna. 3—Compound fracture (bone protrudes through skin). 4—Greenstick fracture. 5—Broken ball of femur.

The broken parts of a bone should be brought back to their natural positions as soon as possible and should be held in place until they have grown together. If a fracture is not attended to, the bones may grow together at an angle, making a crooked leg, for example; or where bones grow together while they are overlapped, the leg will be shorter than normal.

If an injury is not attended to until several hours after it has occurred, swelling may be so great that it is impossible to tell whether there is a fracture, a dislocation or merely a bruise. In such cases it may be necessary to wait several days for the swelling to go down before treatment is begun. However, in the meantime the injured part should be provided with a temporary splint to guard against further injury.

Reduction is Usually Easy

It is usually easy to reduce a fracture, that is, to put the broken bone parts back to where they belong. Exceptions to this

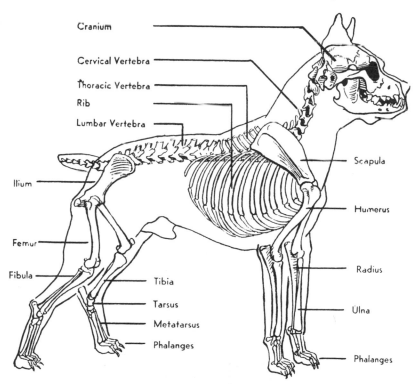

Cranium

Cervical Vertebra

Thoracic Vertebra

Rib

Lumbar Vertebra

Ilium

Femur

Fibula

Tibia

Tarsus

Metatarsus

Phalanges

Scapula

Humerus

Radius

Ulna

Phalanges

101

are where a bone is badly shattered or in cases of broken legs where quite a bit of strength is required to pull against the muscular contractions.

Veterinarians generally put a dog under complete anesthesia before reducing a broken bone. But this should not be done while an animal is suffering from shock which often accompanies an accident, otherwise the animal may die.

After a leg fracture has been reduced, several layers of absorbent cotton should be placed over the affected area and held in place with a bandage. The purpose of this padding is to equalize the pressure of the splints which are placed over it. Splints should be applied in such a way as to hold the broken parts in their normal positions, usually on both sides of a leg. They should be held in place with adhesive tape.

Splints may be made of basswood, veneer, yucca board, cardboard, mailing tubes, wire netting or other rigid or semi-rigid material.

After the swelling has gone down, a permanent cast should be applied. A number of materials are in use for making casts. The more common ones are water glass (sodium silicate), plaster of Paris, and glue.

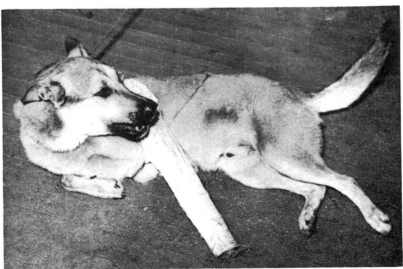

International

Here is a splint made from a large mailing tube. In case of compound fracture, a "window" should be made where the bone has broken through the skin. This permits treatment of the wound in case of infection.

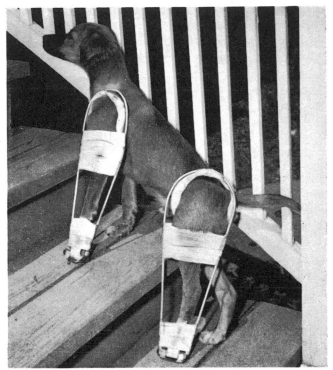

Wearing these specially designed splints even permits a dog to climb stairs, despite two broken legs.

Water glass is light, waterproof, easy to apply and inexpensive, but it irritates the skin and is hard to remove. To apply it, dip strips of muslin, two or three inches wide, into the water glass and bandage the fractured parts with them. Glue is used in a similar way. However, glue is more difficult to apply and has the further disadvantage of drying slowly.

The Plaster of Paris Bandage

Before applying a plaster of Paris bandage to a leg, wrap a few layers of absorbent cotton around the area of the fracture. Hold this in place with a wrapping of cheese cloth or other light material. The layer of cotton should extend both below and above the area to which the plaster bandage is to be applied. This is done to protect the leg against direct contact with the rough edges of the cast.

Use regular plaster of Paris bandages. Put one in water until it is soaked through, that is, until the bubbles stop rising from it. Hold the free end of the bandage in place on the leg with one hand and start wrapping it carefully in a spiral around the leg, unwinding the bandage from the roll as you wind it on the leg.

Each layer of bandage should overlap about half of the preceding one. Should the plaster form roughly or in ridges, smooth it out with a moistened hand. As one roll of bandage is used up, place another in water without delay. Four or five layers of bandage should be applied.

Upon completion of the wrapping, moisten the cast, sprinkle it with plaster of Paris and smooth it out with a moistened hand. The cast will harden in about ten minutes. During that time, the dog, of course, should not be permitted to move.

A cast should be perfectly comfortable. If it is not, then it has either been improperly applied or the fracture was not properly reduced. A leg in a cast must be watched so that a possible infection may be treated immediately.

It takes from three to six weeks for a dog to recover from a fracture, depending upon the age of the animal. During that time, the cast should remain in place. It can be removed by softening it with vinegar and then cutting it way with a razor blade or scissors, being careful not to cut the flesh.

The principles underlying the treatment of all fractures are the same: Bring the broken parts of the bone back to their natural position and keep them there until they grow together. Seldom are two breaks exactly alike. Initiative is often necessary to provide the proper splints and casts.

Bone Dislocations

IT IS SOMETIMES too hard to tell a dislocation from a fracture. In both there is deformity and pain. However in a fracture there is an unnatural mobility of the bone whereas in a dislocation the bone is more or less rigidly fixed in one position. If a bone is broken there is a grating sound when the ends of the bones are rubbed against each other; in a dislocation the injury is in the joint and no such sound occurs when the bone is moved.

The setting of a fracture may be delayed for hours or even several days without harm, but a dislocated joint should be attended to at once. The longer the delay, the greater the damage.

The Most Common Dislocation

The most common dislocation among dogs is nearly always the result of the animal being hit by an automobile. Veterinarians refer to the injury as a "coxofemoral luxation." This means that the dog has had his hip knocked out of joint.

The most frequent form of this dislocation is when the

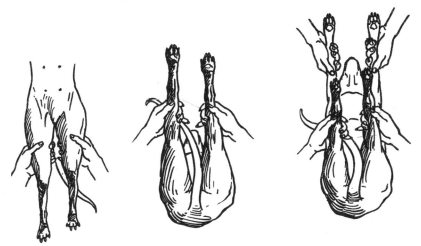

How to tell a dislocated hip: Left—When the legs are stretched backward, the one that is dislocated is shorter. Center—When the legs are held at right angles to the body, the dislocated one is shorter. Right—When the legs are stretched forward, the dislocated one is longer.

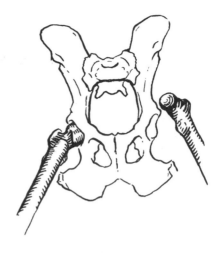

The extreme right of this drawing shows how the ball of the upper leg bone, or femur, is thrown out of its socket with a dislocation.

rounded upper end of the femur is thrown out of its socket, forward and upward. In such cases there is an enlargement that can be felt in front of the normal position of the joint. The leg is fixed in a backward position and the dog refuses to put weight on it. Occasionally the ball of the femur is thrown upward and backward with the enlargement in back of the joint. The limb is then fixed forward and inward.

If possible a dog should be placed under an anesthetic before an attempt is made to treat a dislocated hip. Treatment is painful and a struggling dog is often hard to handle. By feeling the head of the bone and comparing its position with the corresponding bone on the dog's other side, it is easy to tell which way pressure should be exerted to force the head of the bone back into its socket. Both pulling and twisting of the bone are necessary. Some cases are obstinate and with large dogs great strength is sometimes needed by operator.

Dislocation of Shoulder

A dislocation of the shoulder joint does not occur often and when it does it is usually accompanied with a fracture of the humerus, the upper bone of the front leg. The dislocation can easily be recognized by feeling of the shoulder and comparing it with the one on the other side. The bone will usually go back into place if one person holds the dog firmly while another gives the upper leg a sharp pull forward.

Elbow Dislocations

In a dislocation at the elbow, the head of the radius may be displaced inwardly or outwardly. The joint appears immovable, and enlarged. There is much pain and lameness.

To treat this dislocation, the upper limb should be held firmly by an assistant. The operator should then pull the lower leg downward and across the opposite leg and hold it firmly in that position, while the fingers of the other hand press the head of the displaced bone back into its normal position.

In this dislocation, the large retaining ligament has been ruptured or strained and the bone will again slip out of place if the dog stands on the leg. For this reason a plaster bandage is necessary to hold the bones in place until the strained or ruptured ligaments have healed.

Dislocated Knee Cap

The joint that corresponds to the knee of humans is called the stifle joint. As with humans it has a patella, otherwise known as a kneecap.

A dislocated kneecap occurs often in Boston Terriers, less often in Pomeranians, Pekingese, and Japanese Spaniels. Like other dislocations, it is painful. The animal holds his leg in a bent position and refrains from walking on the affected leg. Diagnosis is usually easy since the kneecap is out of place.

To reduce this dislocation, draw the leg backward and straighten it out as much as possible; then force the bone back into place with the fingers. Sometimes a dislocated kneecap becomes chronic in which case veterinarians may perform a difficult operation involving a ligament.

INDEX

A

Abdomen—
 enlargement of, 9
 fluid in, 67
 tender, 9
 abnormal growths and swellings, 83–90
Abscesses, 83
 how to treat, *pictures* 87
Acid poisoning, 35–36
Acne, 59
Alkali poisoning, 36
Alopecia (baldness), 60
Alternaria tenuis, 57
Amino acids, necessary for health, 22
Ancylostoma braziliense, 46
Ancylostoma caninum, 46
Anemia—
 caused by worms, 39, 43, 46
 common symptom, 10
 from improper diet, 28–29
Anesthetics, 95–96
Antidotes for poisons, 32–36
Appetite—
 abnormally large, 9
 depraved, 9, 70
 lack of, 9
Arsenic poisoning, 33
Artificial respiration, 96
Ascarids (roundworms), 37–40
Ascites (dropsy), 67

B

Balanced ration, 21–25
Baldness, 60
Bandages—
 after Caesarian operation, *pic-ture* 76
 for ear injuries, *picture* 85
 plaster of Paris, 103
 to stop bleeding, 72
Bee stings, how to treat, 74
Benign tumors, 85–86
Bitches. *See* Nursing bitches, pregnant bitches
Bites, how to treat, 73
Blacktongue, 31

Bleeding, how to stop, 72
Bloat, how to treat, 77
Blood blisters, 84
Boils, 83
Bonemeal, to prevent rickets, 27
Bones—
 fractures, 100–104
 out of joint, 105–107
Brain inflammation (encephalitis), 12
Breath, foul, 9
Breathing, difficult, 9
Burns, how to treat, 74

C

Calcium deficiency—
 eclampsia, 29
 rickets, 27–28
Cancer, 85–86
Canine leptospirosis, 80–81
Canine typhus, 31, 71
Canker of the ear, 65–66
Car sickness, how to treat, 76–77
Carbohydrates, necessary for health, 22–23
Carcinoma, 85–86
Casts, 104
Cataract, 62
Catarrhal gastroenteritis, 70–71
Chloroform, 95
Choking, how to treat, 77
Chorea, aftereffect of distemper, 12
Coccidiosis, 78
Collars, to keep dogs from licking wounds, *pictures* 75
Comminuted fracture, 100
Compound fracture, 100
Conjunctivitis, 61
Constipation, how to treat, 70
Contagious diseases—
 distemper, 11–14
 pink eye, 62
 ringworm, 58–59
Convulsions, 10
Copper deficiency (anemia), 28–29
Coughing, 10
Cropping ears, 92–94
Cuts, how to treat, 73
Cysts, 83–84

108

D

110

Piroplasmosis, 79-80
Plaster of Paris bandage, 103
Pleurisy, 67-68
Pneumonia, 68-69
Poisons—
list of common, 33-36
salmon poisoning, 78-79
Powders, how to give, 99
Pregnant bitches—
eclampsia, 29
feeding, 23
need calcium, 29
need iron, 29
should be dewormed, 145
Proteins, necessary for health, 22
Prussic acid poisoning, 36
Pulse—
how to take, 7-8, *picture* 7
normal, 7
Puppies—
docking tails, 91-92
feeding, 22, 23, 25

R

Rabies, 18-20
Rectum, itchy, 65
Red mange, 50-51
Removing objects from throat, 77
Rickets, 27-28
Ringworm, 58-59
Rocky Mountain spotted fever, 55
Roundworms, 37-40
trichinosis, 82
Rules of feeding, 25-26
Running fits, 63
Rupture, 89-90

S

St. Vitus dance, aftereffect of distemper, 12
Salmon poisoning, 78-79
Salt—
as an emetic, 32
in food, 23
Sarcoptic mange, 51-52
Scabies, 51-52
Scalds, how to treat, 74
Scrotal hernia, 89-90
Secondary infections, following distemper, 12
Sedatives, to control spasms, 34
Shock, how to treat, 73-74
Simple fracture, 100

Skin diseases—
acne, 59
dandruff, 60
eczema, 57-58
mange, 50-53
ringworm, 58-59
Skin disturbances, 10
Slobbering, 10
Snake bit, how to treat, 74, 76
Spasms, controlled by sedatives, 34
Spleen, enlargement of, 86
Splints, 102
Sticktight fleas, 56, *picture* 56
Stings, how to treat, 74
Stomach, how to puncture, 77
Strychnine poisoning, 34
Stuttgart disease, 31, 71
Summer itch, 57-58
Suppurative keratitis, 61-62
Swellings—
abnormal, 83-90
common symptom, 10
Symptoms—
list of common, 9-10
three kinds, 4

T

Tablets, how to give, 99
Tails, how to dock, 91-92
Tapeworms, 44-45
Temperature—
how to take, 6
normal, 5
Thermometer, how to use, 6
Thiamin (vitamin B1), 30
Thirst, abnormal, 10
Throat, removing objects from, 77
Ticks, 54-55, *pictures* 54, 55
cause piroplasmosis, 79-80
Tongue, coated, 10
Tourniquet, to stop bleeding, 72
Toxascaris canis, 38
Toxascaris leonina, 38
Trembling, 10
Trichinosis, 82
Tularemia, 55
Tumors, 84-86

U

Umbilical hernia, 89
Uncinaria stenocephala, 46
Underfeeding, 25

V

Vaccination—
  for distemper, 14
  for hard pad disease, 17
  for infectious hepatitis, 16
  for rabies, 20
Virus diseases—
  distemper, 11-14
  hard pad disease, 16-17
  infectious hepatitis, 15-16
  rabies, 18-20
Vitamins, necessary for health, 22, 27-31
Vomiting, 10

W

Warts, 86, 88

Wasp stings, how to treat, 74
Weaning—
  age for, 22
  feeding before and after, 22, 23, 25
Weight—
  feed required, per pound, 25
  loss of, 10
  two methods for weighing, *pictures*, 24
Weil's disease, 80
Whipworms, 42-44
Worms, 37-49

X

Xeropthalmia, 30

RECOMMENDED READING

AFGHAN, HOW TO RAISE AND TRAIN, by Sunny Shay and Sara M. Barbaresi, 64 pp., $1.00. Profusely illustrated, covering breeding through adulthood. One of TFH series including *How to Raise and Train an Airedale, Akita, American Foxhound, American Water Spaniel, Basset, Beagle, Bedlington Terrier, Bloodhound, Border Terrier, Borzoi, Brittany Spaniel, Cairn Terrier, Chesapeake Bay Retriever, Coonhound, Curlycoat Retriever, Dachshund, Dandie Dinmont, English Cocker, English Foxhounds, English Setter, German Shorthaired Pointer, Golden Retriever, Gordon Setter, Irish Setter, Irish Terrier, Irish Water Spaniel, Labrador Retriever, Norwegian Elkhound, Otterhound, Pointer, Rhodesian Ridgeback, Scottish Deerhound, Vizsla, Weimaraner* and *Welsh Terrier*, all $1.00 each.

AFGHAN HOUND, THIS IS THE, by Joan Brearley, 223 pp., History, Standards, Breeding Care and Showing covered and illustrated. One of TFH series including *This is the Beagle, Cocker Spaniel, Dachshund, Labrador Retriever, Poodle,* and *Weimaraner*.

BREED YOUR DOG, by Dr. Leon Whitney, 64 pp., $1.00. Instructive photos in color and black and white, covering breeding through puppyhood.

DOG OWNER'S ENCYCLOPEDIA OF VETERINARY MEDICINE, by Allan H. Hart, B.V.Sc., 186 pp., $9.95. A treatise on canine diseases, their causes, symptoms and treatments.

DOLLARS IN DOGS, by Leon F. Whitney, D.V.M., 255 pp. Twenty-six chapters on vocations in the dog world.

FIRST AID FOR YOUR DOG, by Dr. Herbert Richards, 64 pp., $1.00. Illustrations in color and black and white.

GROOM YOUR DOG, by Leon F. Whitney, D.V.M., 64 pp., $1.00. Illustrations in color and black and white on various grooming techniques.

HOW TO FEED YOUR DOG, by Dr. Leon F. Whitney, 64 pp., $1.00. Diets and feeding routines for puppies and dogs, with illustrations.

HOW TO HOUSEBREAK AND TRAIN YOUR DOG, by Arthur Liebers, 80 pp., $1.00. Six educational chapters illustrated in color and black and white.

HOW TO RAISE AND TRAIN A PEDIGREED OR MIXED BREED PUPPY, by Arthur Liebers, 64 pp., $1.00. Nine chapters on choosing your puppy and breeding it. Illustrated in color and black and white.

HOW TO SHOW YOUR DOG, by Virginia Tuck Nichols, 252 pp., $4.95. For the novice who wants to show his dog.

HUNTING WITH FLUSHING DOGS, by Joe Stetson, 64 pp., $1.00. Illustrated text on training spaniels to flush and retrieve game. One of a series of TFH Publications, including *Hunting with Pointing Dogs, Hunting with Retrievers,* and *Hunting with Scent Hounds,* all $1.00 each.

All books published by TFH Publications, 211 West Sylvania Ave., Neptune City, NJ 07753, and available at pet shops everywhere. Titles not quickly obtainable locally can be ordered from the publisher; in such cases, please add 50c per copy to cover postage and handling.

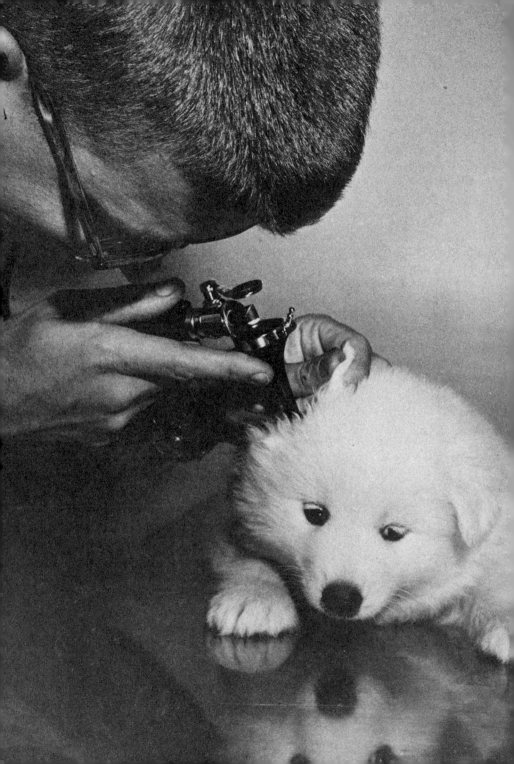

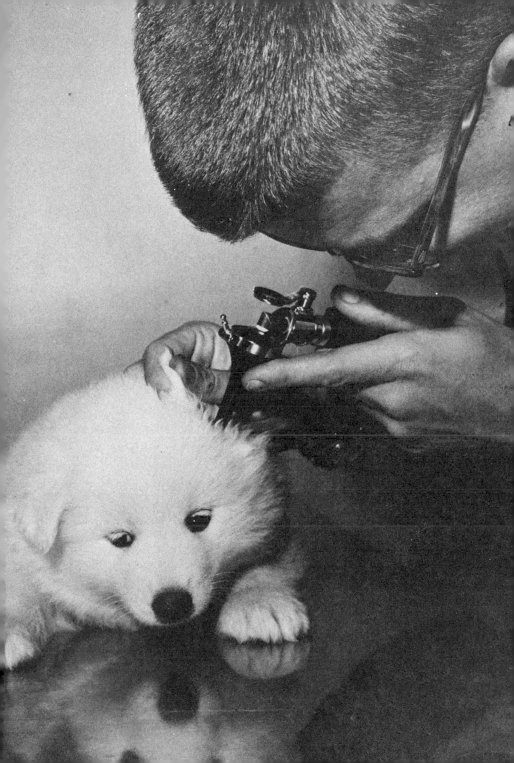

DOG OWNERS VETERINARY GUIDE
AP-927